The ADHD Fraud

ഇൗ ൙

How Psychiatry Makes "Patients"
of Normal Children

ഇൗ ൙

Fred A. Baughman, Jr., M.D.
&
Craig Hovey

Note for Librarians: A cataloguing record for this book is available from Library and Archives Canada at www.collectionscanada.ca/amicus/index-e.html
ISBN 1-4120-6458-9

Printed in Victoria, BC, Canada. Printed on paper with minimum 30% recycled fibre. Trafford's print shop runs on "green energy" from solar, wind and other environmentally-friendly power sources.

TRAFFORD
PUBLISHING™
Offices in Canada, USA, Ireland and UK
This book was published *on-demand* in cooperation with Trafford Publishing. On-demand publishing is a unique process and service of making a book available for retail sale to the public taking advantage of on-demand manufacturing and Internet marketing. On-demand publishing includes promotions, retail sales, manufacturing, order fulfilment, accounting and collecting royalties on behalf of the author.

Book sales for North America and international:
Trafford Publishing, 6E–2333 Government St.,
Victoria, BC v8t 4p4 CANADA
phone 250 383 6864 (toll-free 1 888 232 4444)
fax 250 383 6804; email to orders@trafford.com
Book sales in Europe:
Trafford Publishing (uk) Limited, 9 Park End Street, 2nd Floor
Oxford, UK oxi ihh UNITED KINGDOM
phone 44 (0)1865 722 113 (local rate 0845 230 9601)
facsimile 44 (0)1865 722 868; info.uk@trafford.com
Order online at:
trafford.com/05-1369

10 9 8 7

DEDICATIONS

This book is dedicated to parents and children everywhere—all of them told the "chemical imbalance" lie and drugged. None can imagine a betrayal so deceitful, so complete, by educators, psychologists, psychiatrists, pediatricians, neurologists, family practitioners, the pharmaceutical industry, the White House, the Senate, the House of Representatives and all agents and agencies of government. When a child has been killed or maimed by a drug, made a drug addict, a crazed killer, or a suicide, or when a parent sees custody of their child—their flesh and blood—given the parent who plays psychiatry's game, or to the court itself—which always does—they awake, too late, to the fact that the betrayal has been complete, that there was never a disease to treat, never a "chemical imbalance" to balance—that ADHD and all psychiatric "diseases" were a total, 100% fraud all along.

—Fred A. Baughman, Jr. & Craig Hovey

I wish to dedicate this book to my co-author, Dr. Fred Baughman, a man of unmatched integrity, compassion, and courage.

—Craig Hovey

To Craig Hovey, for understanding from the start the totality of the fraud of psychiatry's invented "diseases"/"chemical imbalances"—and for helping me say it clearly and unflinchingly.

—Fred A. Baughman, Jr., M.D.

Acknowledgement

In our home, the buck stops with my wife, Annette I. Baughman, mother of our three children. That she would cede responsibility for her family to no one served us well in 1970, when educators sought to label and drug the older of our two sons. Annette attended his classes and found a dedicated teacher, Miss Jones, who volunteered to take him in her class, convinced, as were we, that he could behave and learn appropriate to his age and grade level without psychiatric or pharmacological intervention. Today that son owns his own political consultancy and is a success on the national scene, our daughter is a successful criminal defense attorney, loving wife, and mother of two of our three wonderful grandchildren, and our youngest son is a brilliant engineer and loving father to the third of our grandchildren, a daughter. A mother's instincts can provide immunity to ADHD and to many of the worlds maladies and pitfalls. Annette has been affording me such protection for 45 years. I know.

Love,
Your husband—Fred

Contents

Chapter One—A CHILDREN'S CRUSADE   1
1. Deputy Diagnosticians: You've Got
   "Ants In The Pants"
2. 100% Fraud
3. Stephanie's Story
4. The Disappearing Boy
5. No Tolerance For Normal
6. Anger Rising
7. A Widening Plague
8. The Real Villian

Chapter Two—MAKING MONKEYS   22
1. The Making Of Monkeys
2. The Big Con
3. A Shock To The System
4. A Neurologist's Nightmare
5. No Difference Allowed
6. Treating Normal Behavior As Abnormal
7. The Boy Who Was Mistaken For A Monkey
8. A Collective Madness
9. Statement Of Patricia Weathers

Chapter Three—EVOLUTION OF AN EPIDEMIC:
A DRUG IN SEARCH OF A DISEASE   52
1. A Drug In Search Of A Disease
2. Preview Of The Plague
3. Back To The Future
4. From Attacks On Individual Children
   To An Attack On Childhood Itself
5. Drugs R Us: A Pill For Every Child

Chapter Four—DOLLARS FOR DISEASES   75
  1. Dollars For Diseases
  2. Death By Desipramine: Shaina's Story
  3. What Is A Disease?
  4. How A Real Disease Is Discovered And Verified
  5. The Making Of Psychopharmacology:
    How Money Fuels The Invasion Of
    Psychiatry Into Daily Life

Chapter Five—THE DSM: DANGEROUSLY STRANGE
                 MANEUVERS   102

Chapter Six—ATTACK OF THE PAPER PUSHERS   140
  1. Attack Of The Paper Pushers
  2. The Devil In Black And White
  3. Not Just For Kids Anymore
  4. ADD In Adults
  5. The Marketing Of Mental Illness

Chapter Seven—SCIENCE FOR SALE   165
  1. Doctored Deceit
  2. The Erosion Of Government Protection
  3. Smoke And Mirrors
  4. Induce Brain Atrophy, Call It A Disease
  5. Genetics Claims
  6. Mri Brain Scans In Adhd (Always Treated)
  7. Swanson & Castellanos Seek To Prove
    ADHD A Disease
  8. Still Refusing To Do Valid Research
  9. A Confession: No Such Thing As
    A Psychiatric Disease
  10. Spinning A Web Of Deceit
  11. Lying To Patients—the New Standard Of Practice

Chapter Eight—PUSHING POISONS   189
1. Pushing Poisons
2. Daniel In The Lion's Den
3. The Right (& Duty) Of Informed Consent
4. Getting Off Psychiatric Drugs

Chapter Nine—IMMUNIZE YOUR CHILD AGAINST ADHD 203
1. Not A Disease—Just A Normal Child
2. The First Line Of Defense: The Schools
3. Be An Assertive Parent/Guardian
4. Rational Suspicion
5. The Predators Among Us
6. A Tightening Noose
7. A Wide Range Of Normal

Chapter Ten—AFTERWORD   218
1. I (FB) Testify To The Parliament Of
   Western Australia
2. Do Not Allow Testing Or Labeling:
   The Only Absolute Immunity

Chapter Eleven—ALERT!   226
1. Adderall causes 20 deaths and 12 strokes!

ENDNOTES   234

INDEX   265

FOREWORD

by

Martin Whitely B. Com. Dip. Ed. JP MLA

Member of the Legislative Assembly
Parliament of Western Australia

ADHD was not discovered by science, it was voted into existence in 1987 by a committee of the American Psychiatric Association. Beginning with that vote a series of political processes have resulted in widespread international recognition of ADHD as a "psychiatric disorder".

Medicine and psychiatry are supposed to be driven by hard science, not politics supported by pseudo-science. ADHD has snowballed internationally because the outrageous claims of the ADHD industry have often escaped scrutiny.

As a result, across the globe over the last 15 years, millions of responsible loving parents have accepted at face value the advice of an "expert" child psychiatrist or pediatrician and "medicated" their child for ADHD.

Typically these parents have been told their child has a biochemical imbalance in the brain best treated with safe effective stimulant medication.

Most are never told the truth.

Most are never told that there is no proof of a biochemical imbalance in their child's brain.

Most are never told that their child's diagnosis of ADHD is entirely based on second hand reports of their child's behavior.

Most are never told the diagnostic criteria are no more objective than a teacher's observation that their child avoids homework, interrupts, fidgets, squirms in their seat, loses pens and pencils, and is forgetful and disorganized.

None are ever shown a blood test or a brain scan or any scientific proof of their child's supposed chemical imbalance of the brain. Why? Because they don't exist.

Most are never told that the amphetamines used to treat ADHD are drugs of addiction with a startling range of adverse side effects and unknown long-term effects on developing minds and bodies.

These parents are denied their right to informed consent about their child's treatment.

Many children are naturally inattentive, impulsive and hyperactive. In these cases normal behavior is pathologized and normal, healthy children are drugged.

Some children, however, do have a range of real problems that cause disruptive behavior. For example, children who can't hear or see properly may be inattentive or impulsive because they are frustrated with not being able to keep up with the rest of the class. Likewise, children not taught to read properly and children traumatized by events beyond their control. It is hardly surprising that drugging these children with behavior- altering amphetamines alters their behavior, masking the symptoms but doing nothing to deal with the underlying cause.

An Australian boy, Brandon's story is disturbing but typical of too many children worldwide. Brandon had been first medicated for behavioral problems when he was 4. By early 2004 Brandon (then 12) was on Dexamphetamine for ADHD, Sodium Valproate for mood stabilization, and tranquilizers to calm him down. Brandon suffered mood swings, migraines, insomnia and sleepwalking, chronic stomachaches, and was unnaturally thin.

A residential intensive intervention program turned around Brandon and his family's life. Brandon was initially detoxified and his mother Katherine participated in effective parenting sessions. Brandon's real problems—hearing and learning difficulties—were identified. Brandon is now drug free, happy, well-behaved (for a 13 year old boy), and with extra in-class support he is performing well academically.

Virtually all the symptoms of ADHD relate to classroom behavior. Children who don't do homework, fidget, squirm, interrupt, and are forgetful and disorganized are assumed to have a biochemical imbalance in their brain.

These children can be difficult to control in a classroom and in many cases are more compliant when drugged. However, there is absolutely no scientifically valid evidence that compliant-drugged students learn faster.

There may be an argument for drugging psychotic adults who represent a danger to others but there is absolutely no justification for drugging children to keep them quiet. Surely it is a basic right of every child to grow up free from unnecessary biochemical interference.

ADHD is a "disorder" manufactured to match our times. It is a quick catch-all diagnosis with a magic bullet treatment. The contrived ADHD epidemic started in the United States and has been adopted around the globe with varying degrees of enthusiasm.

My home Perth, Western Australia has the highest prescription rates of amphetamines in Australia. Western Australian children are 4 times more likely than other Australian children to be diagnosed ADHD and drugged with amphetamines. In 2002 Western Australia per-head prescription rates first exceeded the USA national average.

Do Perth children have different brain chemistry from children in Sydney, San Diego, Chicago or London? Of course they don't. The real difference isn't in the brain chemistry or behavior of these children but rather in the clinical practice of the pediatricians and child psychiatrists who treat them.

Perth with a population of 1.5 million is one of the most isolated cities in the world. It has one medical school and a closed medical community who are reluctant to criticize each other.

This lack of a critical culture allowed a handful of irresponsible clinicians to diagnose and drug without proper scrutiny. It was only the intervention of a parliamentary committee of the Western Australian Parliament that turned the debate in Perth.

Ironically, it was Perth's politicians who reminded Perth's medical fraternity that medical practice should follow science not fashion.

Dr. Baughman's testimony to the parliamentary committee was crucial in exposing the scientific fraud that underpins ADHD. On a personal level Fred gave me some very sound advice in dealing with the ADHD industry "experts."

He said that when asked for proof of the existence of ADHD, "experts" will typically respond there are hundreds of scientific papers validating ADHD. However, when asked which report confirms the existence of an objective physical abnormality making ADHD a disease, psychiatry cannot identify a single such report.

I followed Dr. Baughman's advice and he was right. Good science isn't about quantity of research, it is however about facts. None of the hundreds of papers sited by the ADHD industry prove ADHD is an actual disease or that amphetamines are a safe and effective treatment.

As a substitute for real evidence the ADHD industry presents "consensus statements" or even "internationally consensus statements" of "ADHD experts" who all sign a document devoid of scientific substance but concluding unanimously that ADHD is real and common.

Like the fabled adulation of the Emperor's New Clothes, the growth of and enthusiasm for ADHD ignores the blindingly obvious.

In the minds of the medical profession, politicians and policy makers, ADHD has got so big it must be real. But like the emperor's new clothes ADHD has no substance.

Dr. Baughman is filling the role of the boy who pointed out that the Emperor was naked. He has reminded us that children are inattentive, impulsive, and hyperactive and that amphetamines are addictive and dangerous.

Fred Baughman has exposed ADHD and the industry it has spawned for what it is. Fraud.

Chapter One

A CHILDREN'S CRUSADE

We are witnessing a crisis of a magnitude and type never seen before.

- William Carey M.D.

On the afternoon of March 21, 2000, fourteen-year-old Matthew Smith was having a good time in his aunt's basement, skateboarding with two of his cousins. Suddenly he fell off the skateboard and collapsed to the floor, where his frightened cousins say he started moaning and turned blue. Paramedics were called immediately but were unable to revive him. Matthew was taken to Royal Oak William Beaumont hospital where he was pronounced dead.

The fall did not kill Matthew. According to an autopsy by Dr. Ljubisa Dragovic, the teenager had died of a heart attack—a heart attack caused by Ritalin. The Death Certificate fingered the best known of the drugs prescribed to treat attention deficit/ hyperactivity disorder (ADHD), "Death caused from long term use of Methylphenidate (Ritalin)," it read. Matthew had started taking the drug at the age of seven after being diagnosed with ADHD. After eight years of it, his life was over.

Because the death was sudden, with no cause apparent at first, Dr. Dragovic, chief pathologist of the Oakland County Medical Examiner's Office in Michigan, was called in to perform an autopsy. He discovered that the small blood vessels that fed Matthew's heart had been scarred and grown thicker, and that the heart itself had sustained damage and become enlarged because it had to work harder to compensate for the impaired vessels. As

Dr. Dragovic told the *Oakland Press*, "This was a gradual development. There were changes that occurred in the small blood vessels that supply the heart muscle." He added that, "Over a period of time, there is a buildup of changes. Finally, these changes get to the point that they become incompatible with life."

Never had Dr. Dragovic witnessed this set of conditions in anybody so young. Usually they are found in adults with a history of abusing stimulants, such as cocaine and amphetamines. [1] [2] But it has become increasingly common now for ADHD-diagnosed children to be given stimulants for long periods of time. Though Ritalin is usually presented as a mild stimulant, it is nearly identical to cocaine and is actually more potent at comparable dosages, something Matthew's parents had no idea of, eight years earlier, when Matthew's school repeatedly insisted that he had ADHD and needed to be given Ritalin.

The Drug Enforcement Administration (DEA) published a background paper on methylphenidate (the generic name for Ritalin) in 1995 [3] that stated, "Methylphenidate is a Schedule II central nervous system stimulant and shares many of the pharmacological effects of amphetamines, metamphetamine, and cocaine." A Schedule II drug is a classification the DEA reserves for the most dangerous and addictive drugs that can be prescribed legally. To educators at Matthew's school, however, Ritalin was simply a magic pill that made troublesome students easier to manage.

What of Matthew's ADHD diagnosis? Is it a disease? Was he a child in dire need of medication, somebody for whom the risks of side effects or even death were outweighed by the benefits of his prescribed drug? His parents, Larry and Kelly, do not think so. Prior to being diagnosed Matthew was an energetic, social child who sometimes was boisterous and did not focus on his school work the way his teachers wanted him to, but this is hardly abnormal for a six-year-old boy.

As Larry tells it, Matthew was a lot like him, his dad, at that age, a kid who liked being actively involved in what he was doing and functioned better outside of the stifling confines of the classroom. Larry speaks of skipping school as a boy and going to a construction site where he would gather up scrap lumber and build a tree house, finding satisfaction in things like this, and music, where he could make use of the talents he possessed, talents that did not always mesh well with school requirements. Larry says that if the ADHD diagnosis were around when he was a child he would have been labeled and drugged, too, just like his son. Yet, neither Larry or Matthew ever had any real problems with paying attention or being hyperactive. They are examples of perfectly normal people who just happened to be a poor fit with the demands and expectations of their school systems, just like most of the millions of the normal children who are being labeled ADHD and forced to take powerful drugs today.

The push to label and drug Matthew began when he was in first grade. School officials said he was fidgety in his seat, would sometimes interrupt the class, and often had trouble staying focused on his work. The school social worker called Larry and Kelly in for repeated meetings where she informed them that Matthew had ADHD and needed to be medicated. If Matthew's school were functioning properly it would have been scandalous for an unqualified social worker to take on the role of physician and make a diagnosis and recommendation for medication. This constitutes practicing medicine without a license, which is illegal. The same, unfortunately, has been done in school districts across the nation by thousands of teachers, administrators, counselors, psychologists, and social workers for years now.

An increasing number of people who work within the educational establishment are deeply disturbed by this practice, like the school psychologist from a large district (approximately 55,000 students) who e-mailed us to say, "I have been horrified by the numbers of children who are put on stimulant medication on the basis of the word of a misguided teacher or administrator. Too many parents report to me that they are told to get their kid on Ritalin or Adderall or they will be placed in special education programs (which do not work, by the way). They are also given the

names of local physicians who serve as stimulant "automats" (the
teacher said it, so it's good enough for me)." This is no small breach
of ethics. Physicians prescribing powerful medication should first
perform a complete physical exam and fully inform the parents of
exactly what the diagnosis means and what the risks of the medication are. Failure to do so, a violation of every patient's right to
informed consent, is grounds for malpractice.

DEPUTY DIAGNOSTICIANS:
YOU'VE GOT "ANTS IN THE PANTS"

In the vast majority of cases it is schools, with the process
usually kicked off by a classroom teacher, who initiate the ADHD
labeling and drugging process, not parents or physicians. Despite
having no qualifications for making diagnoses or recommending
drugs, they are brazen about it. A story that typifies what we hear
from parent after parent comes from the mother who reports that,
"I was told by the first grade teacher that my child suffers from
'ants in the pants.' This same teacher filled out an ADHD evaluation form that the school psychologist looked at, then shared his
conclusion with the mother that "...my child placed in the significant range overall for symptoms of ADHD." Their pediatrician
followed suit and the child was officially diagnosed and put on
Ritalin, with never a better reason emerging than those "ants in
the pants."

Another practice, which has become more common in recent years, is for school officials to threaten parents with reports
to social service agencies if they resist medicating their children
when told to. This very threat was made to Larry and Kelly, who
feared that they could lose custody of their children if they did
not comply. Testifying before the House Education Committee
in 2001, Larry said that, "They were pretty much writing the prescription before he even saw the doctor. We were threatened with
social services if we didn't get him on the medication."

Reluctantly, Larry and Kelly took Matthew to a pediatrician the school recommended for an evaluation. According to Larry the doctor seemed frustrated by the school's diagnosis and push for medication and asked Larry to let the school know that, "I am not a pharmacy." When a prescription did not follow quickly enough the school social worker wrote the doctor a letter to hurry him along. Larry shared a copy of the letter with us, dated November 22, 1991, which contained the following: "We had hoped by September you and Matt's parents would have begun a trial of medication so that we could assess whether his learning would have benefited by increased focus and concentration. Would you consider simultaneously having Matt begin his 3 hours in a resource room with a prescribed medical therapy?"

Ritalin, along with the other popular stimulants prescribed for ADHD, like Dexedrine (dextro-amphetamine) and Adderall (dextroamphetamine saccharate and sulfate; amphetamine aspartate and sulfate), increase just about anybody's focus and concentration. This is why the illegal use of these and similar drugs are popular on high school and college campuses when papers are due and tests loom. As is well documented in the medical literature, however, using speed, uppers, and prescription stimulants, though they may feel like performance boosters in the short run, come with a significant downside that far outweighs any temporary effect. In the letter quoted above, the school social worker is expressing her disapproval of the doctor for not medicating Matt quickly enough and is trying to move him along, also inferring that he is delaying the improvements in school performance sure to come. And those improvements, i.e., a more manageable child, would only be in the school's eyes. No ADHD drug has ever been shown to enhance academic performance over the long term. [4] Her ignorance of what Ritalin really is (as you will see in the pages ahead) served to push Matthew along a fatal path.

Though the stimulant drugs given for ADHD do not benefit the children taking them in any way, they do make "troublesome" kids easier to manage in the here and now. By suppressing some typical behaviors of childhood they cause children to act less like the normal kids they really are and more like the docile adults who are supposed to be teaching them. The following quote from a parent writing to psychologist/columnist John Rosemond in the November 10, 2001 *San Diego Union-Tribune* is an alarming example of what happens in schools throughout the country, "This is my son's first year in a new, private school. Already, his third-grade teacher has suggested that we have him tested for attention deficit disorder. I discovered that 65 (sixty-five) percent of the kids in the fifth grade at his school have been diagnosed with ADD and are taking medication."

Kelly Smith observed that on Ritalin Matt was more subdued, had greater focus, and could better attend to what he was expected to do in school. Such a result is usually pointed to as proof that the child in question really has ADHD, but the truth is that Ritalin and the other ADHD drugs are intended to do nothing more than control unwanted (though normal) behaviors. Dr. Debra Zarin, representing the American Psychiatric Association and the American Academy of Child and Adolescent Psychiatry, testified on July 16, 1996, before a Congressional subcommittee conducting a hearing on federal responses to issues involving the treatment of ADHD, that, "It is a commonly held misconception that if a stimulant calms a child, that he must have ADHD; if he didn't have the disorder, the thinking goes, the medication would not have any effect. That is not true. Stimulants increase attention span in normal children as well as those with ADHD." [5] The only disagreement we have with the above statement is where she refers to "...those with ADHD." As we will show throughout the book, because there is still no evidence to warrant consideration of ADHD as a medical disease, it does not make sense to refer to anybody "with" or "having" ADHD.

As Matt's performance was being "enhanced" his heart was slowly being destroyed, a process the medical examiner called "silent and smoldering," with its existence not known until it was too late. Anabolic steroids will enhance a youngster's performance in the sense that taking them yields greater endurance and larger and more powerful muscles, but should these drugs be administered just because they produce an effect adults consider desirable. [6] Certainly not, for the risks far outweigh the benefits. And the risks of force-feeding drugs like Ritalin do not just consist of unjustifiable physical side effects, but of the damage done by teaching a child that his or her brain cannot work right without drugs, that the child does not possess the capacity to measure up to adult standards without it. Psychiatrist Peter Breggin has said, "...we abuse our children with drugs rather than making the effort to find better ways to meet their needs. In the end, we are giving our children a very bad lesson—that drugs are the answer to emotional problems. We are encouraging a generation of youngsters to grow up relying on psychiatric drugs rather than on themselves and other human resources."

According to Larry, in addition to recommending over and over again that Matt be medicated with Ritalin, "They told us that Ritalin was safe and would help Matthew a lot." Larry and Kelly, like most parents, saw the educators they dealt with as experts and, though they were opposed to medicating their son and did not see him as abnormal at all, succumbed to the school's threats, badgering, and outright misinformation and allowed Matthew to begin taking Ritalin, which their doctor also assured them was safe. They had no idea there were any possible side effects or negative consequences until after he died.

Larry told *The Detroit News* that, "His last report card was his best. But it wasn't worth it for us. Putting him on Ritalin was the worst decision I've ever made." Dr. Dragovic, the medical examiner, told the same newspaper this about Ritalin: "It is a stimulant, a serious medication. It should be considered seriously by parents before it is prescribed for prolonged use. Chronic long-term exposure can lead to a catastrophe like this." In a heartbreaking conversation Larry told us, "If it wasn't for the pressure of the school system, Matt would still be alive today."

100% FRAUD

Between the years 1990 and 2000 the Food and Drug Administration received 186 reports of death caused by methylphenidate (Ritalin and all other forms of the drug) through its MedWatch program, a voluntary system for the reporting of post-marketing complications of drugs. [7] Epidemiological studies have shown that voluntary systems, such as this, report no more than 1 to 10 percent of actual adverse reactions, so the death count for Ritalin is sure to be much higher, as are the totals for the following additional negative effects reported due to methylphenidate: 569 hospitalizations (36 were life-threatening), 949 central or peripheral nervous system occurrences, 126 cardiovascular occurrences, 6 cases of cardiomyopathy, 12 of arrhythmia, 7 of bradycardia (slow pulse), 5 of bundle branch block (impairment of heart's conduction apparatus), 4 of EKG abnormality, 5 extrasystole (heart rhythm abnormalities), 3 of heart arrest, 2 of heart failure, 10 of hypotension (low blood pressure), 1 myocardial infarction (heart attack), and 15 cases of tachycardia (rapid pulse).

Ritalin is just one of the drugs commonly prescribed for ADHD. Why doesn't anybody know the true number of children harmed or killed by Ritalin and other psychiatric drugs? There is no nationwide data-gathering system that allows us to calculate the exact number of Ritalin-induced deaths or damage, or those induced by other psychiatric medications, but it is certain that parents and patients alike are routinely misled and uninformed. Even if the numbers the FDA does have represent only a sliver of the real total, they are still more than enough to raise alarms. The truth is that Ritalin and other psychiatric drugs given to children are dangerous, addictive substances that provide no benefits while exposing them to horrible risks.

The Smiths and millions of other parents have been told that ADHD is a neurological disorder, one that exists just as surely as any physical disease like diabetes or cancer. As our book shows, this is a lie. ADHD is not a disease, disorder, or abnormality that has ever been discovered or verified. Any claims that it has a bio-logical basis are pure speculation with no scientific evidence to back them up. If ADHD was meant as a way merely to identify a set of behaviors with no inference of it being a neurological abnormality, that would be one thing (and still an insult to children), but the insistence that it exists in the same physical and provable realm as real diseases is a perversion of science, without even enough credibility to rise to the level of pseudo science or junk science. It is an outright lie. [8]

What happened to Matthew Smith and his parents is not an isolated case. There are approximately 6 million children in the United States, and many millions more around the world, who have been diagnosed with, and drugged for, ADHD. ADHD has never been objectively identified in a single one of them, not one—and it never will be. ADHD is not a disorder or a disease or a syndrome or a chemical imbalance of the brain, it is not over-diagnosed or under-diagnosed or misdiagnosed. It does not exist in 3% or 5% or 15% of the population. It is a 100% fraud.

To bring home just how devastating this fraud can be, here is the story of Stephanie Hall:

STEPHANIE'S STORY

Stephanie Hall was a fun-loving, outdoorsy girl with a joy for life who tried to make butterflies and ladybugs her pets. She liked to collect acorns, buckeyes, and pine combs and had a love for flowers. She was warm and never quit wanting to hug people, also liking to give family members big kisses on the cheek. Stephanie had two younger sisters she loved very much.

Stephanie Hall lived from January 11, 1984, until January 5, 1996, dying the morning after her Ritalin dosage was upped, a drug she had been taking for five years, beginning soon after her school initiated the process of having her diagnosed for ADD. Her mother says, "I am glad she had a happy childhood outside of school."

As Janet Hall remembers, "In 1st grade Stephanie was a quiet, shy girl. She had a great love of books. She just loved school and made new friends easily. Then, it was about the 2nd or 3rd week of school, her teacher told me that Stephanie had a hard time staying on task and that she was making clicking and humming noises. Sometimes Stephanie would get out of her seat and hug the teacher. She was never a problem at home. She suggested that Stephanie be tested for ADD and said that she could be seen by the school psychologist, at no cost to us."

Though the teacher did not mention any particular drug by name, she did suggest to Stephanie's parents that medication might help. [9]

"We took her to another psychologist instead. He said she was easily distracted but could read just fine and had normal intelligence. Aside from ear infections as a preschooler Steph was healthy as could be, but despite all that she was diagnosed ADD and prescribed Ritalin. It was then that her headaches began...every day, except on weekends, when she didn't take Ritalin."

The Ritalin was initially prescribed by a neurologist the Halls brought her to, with their pediatrician taking over from there. The neurologist based his diagnosis on a 10 minute visit with Stephanie, where he had her read a book and throw a ball, then he read over reports from the psychologist and teacher.

Stephanie's teacher continued to complain about her behavior. The psychologist suggested trying a behavior modification approach, "to deal with some residual effects and strong-willedness," those not taken care of by the Ritalin. Yet, what got modified the most in the days ahead was Stephanie's Ritalin dosage, and it always went up, beginning with 5 mg in the mornings and evenings and eventually increasing to 40 mg a day over the next five years.

When the dosage went up, the school complaints about her behavior would go down, but more disturbing symptoms were also surfacing. Along with the headaches that came during the week, when she was taking Ritalin, she also began complaining of nausea and stomachaches, then came the mood swings and bizarre behavior, along with her neurologist noticing incoordination during his exams of her.

Janet recalls an incident in the 5th grade when, "Stephanie took off running from the child care center she went to after school. The daycare workers chased her but couldn't catch her. She yelled, 'I'm ten-and-a-half now!' She took off across a busy 5-lane road, bought her grandmother a paper and took it all the way downtown where she worked. The daycare workers were screaming at her to come to them. They called me at work. I never worked after school hours again."

One day the following summer when Stephanie was off medication she suddenly "zoned out," according to her mother, and seemed "disconnected." Stephanie told her she loved her. They always told each other this, so Janet thought nothing of it. But then Stephanie said it again, and she had an empty stare on her face.

"Steph, what's the matter?" asked Janet.

"I see her again," replied Stephanie.

"Who?"

"The angel, she looks mad."

Then Stephanie snapped out of it. She said the angel had white and red all around her. Some of the angels were blue, and they all had four wings. Janet shares that "It reminded me of when she was first put on Ritalin back in the 1st and 2nd grade and told me of seeing angels then."

Janet remembers 6th grade beginning with promise.

"Stephanie made friends easily. Her teachers thought she was the greatest. She had a great deal of compassion for others and wanted to help those in need. When she grew up she wanted to be a firefighter and a paramedic and always said, 'Mom I want to save people.' There was a boy she liked. She was doing okay until the day in October when the vice-principal called and said she was swearing, which was totally out of character for Stephanie. She was always a good girl. I had never heard her swear. Some girl had tried to take her lunch money. A few weeks later I caught her swearing at a boy after school let out. I was shocked; I grounded her. Then, her grades started going down, mostly Ds."

By the end of December Janet became so concerned that she asked to have Stephanie's medication increased. Their pediatrician agreed to increase the dose to 25 mg in the morning and 15 mg at noon, beginning after Christmas vacation.

Janet recalls that, "Stephanie returned to school and took the increase that morning. She seemed real weird, out of it. I kept asking, 'Steph, are you okay?' She kept saying, 'I'm okay mom, I'm okay.'"

And when Janet picked her up after school Stephanie did seem okay, not spaced out like she had been in the morning. The rest of the day went smoothly and when Stephanie went to bed she was in a playful mood, as Janet remembers, "She was upstairs jumping around with her littlest sister, asking for a dollar. I said 'It's 9:00 Steph, get to bed. She said, 'Okay mom, I love you.' I love you too, I said."

The next morning Stephanie's dad went into her room to wake her up for school. There was no response. Stephanie had died during the night.

"We called paramedics and the police. Some of them were about to cry. Stephanie was so cold. I kept saying to them, 'She is supposed to bury me, not me bury her.' No other family should know the agony of burying their child."

The coroner ruled death by natural causes, with the cause of Stephanie's death being cardiac arrhythmia. But was it a natural death? Her parents don't think so. Today, the family continues to visit Stephanie's grave frequently. Janet told us, "Before she died she spoke of seeing angels, now she is one."

* * *

Did Ritalin kill Stephanie Hall? She had no preexisting heart problems or any other physical condition that results in this kind of death. When everything else is ruled out, Ritalin remains as the most likely variable. The only significant change that occurred just prior to her death was the increase in the amount of Ritalin she took.

For children with real diseases medication is often given that comes with risks, even the risk of death. These risks are acceptable if the benefits to be had clearly exceed the risks and those making the decision for treatment are fully informed of both. In Stephanie's case, she was given a dangerous medication for a disease that does not exist; never were her parents informed of the purely speculative (at best) nature of ADHD or the true risks of Ritalin. Their right of informed consent, basic to the ethical practice of medicine, was violated, just as it is whenever a parent is told their child suffers from a neurological abnormality (ADHD) that is, in fact, nothing but a fake disease conjured up for profit.

We suppose the argument could be made that the school had no idea of how badly Ritalin was affecting Stephanie and never would have pushed it had they been aware. Maybe.

But wasn't the prescribing doctor aware of the risks, of the fact that ADHD is an unproven creation? The sad reality is that children are all too likely to be attended by physicians who have left their scientific training behind and accepted the myth of ADHD, and are blind to, or willing to accept, both the risks and lack of benefits that come with the prescriptions they write.

A further unfortunate truth is that far too many schools will continue promoting drug use, and even increasing the amount of drugs a child is taking, despite knowing that serious side effects are being experienced—and the prescribing physicians go right along. We hear this over and over again from parents. The real goal is to turn children into compliant sheep sitting quietly in their seats, and schools would much rather let the sheep suffer than be inconvenienced by any who might kick up their heels when free of drugs.

The piece below was written by a mother who went (and is still going) through hell over the ADHD diagnosis and subsequent drugging of her son. Though we did some slight editing, these are her words. This is not an unusual case. We chose to put it here because it is representative of what happens with regularity across the country, from the bullying of the school to the side effects suffered by the child. The names have been changed due to the family's concerns about repercussions from the school.

THE DISAPPEARING BOY

We were told by our son's doctor that Adam might have ADHD, but he was not sure. Shortly after Adam started kindergarten his teacher started saying he wouldn't sit still and asked if we'd had him evaluated for ADHD. When I told her that Adam may or may not have it she said she definitely saw it in him. This is coming from a teacher, not a doctor. How would she know?

The school kept insisting he was ADHD so I brought Adam back to his doctor, who put him on Dexedrine. To us, this made him a totally different child. He was weepy and very emotional and stopped eating. [10] Adam lost so much weight that we kept bringing him back to the doctor. Even though we thought he'd lost too much weight, the doctor said it was okay, he was fine. I hated it. Well, that school year ended and he was passed to the first grade.

I took him off all meds for the whole summer vacation and tried sending him back to school in the fall with a different teacher and on no meds. They kept telling me I needed to put him back on, constantly calling me and sending home notes, so I took him back to the doctor. Adam was put back on the same drug, Dexedrine, after we'd got him back to looking normal with his weight. He lost it all again. The teacher kept calling and telling me Adam needed his dosage upped and that I needed to have it done. Even the school nurse said the same thing. They haunted me until I did. He lost more weight and started having trouble sleeping, so he was given Clonidine [11] to take at bedtime, which helps him sleep.

Okay, fine, they give it a couple months then start up again about upping his meds again. This time I refuse; he'd lost too much weight and was getting depressed. They tried to keep him back in the first grade but I would not let them, so they tried to put him in special ed classes. He passed the test they gave with scores higher than 95% of his peers. They could not put him in special ed classes and were upset at that. The school year finally came to an end.

Again, no meds all summer. He was fine and acted like a normal, healthy little boy. He then started second grade. I again attempted no meds and this time the teacher only started up on the meds being needed because she was told by the school nurse that Adam had ADHD. So again we went back to his doctor. He was going to give him the Dexedrine again but I said no way; he loses too much weight and gets too weepy and depressed. The doctor recommended we try Ritalin. We had heard bad stories about kids on Ritalin so me and my husband asked him tons of questions, like are there any side effects? He said no, that it worked great. We tried it and it was working good, but the teachers still were not happy. They wanted the dosage higher so they pushed and pushed until it was upped. To me, my son seemed to be getting depressed on it but did not lose weight. The doctor decided not to up it again but to try the new drug, Concerta, which was given at a higher dosage than what he was taking on Ritalin. Adam took it for two weeks before I refused to give it to him because he'd lost twelve pounds in the two weeks on it and was seriously depressed.

Even the teacher said the Concerta did nothing for him and to switch him back to Ritalin. We did, and it still was not good enough for them. They are going to keep Adam back in school this year, which I will allow, but I did stop all his meds after reading more about the problems with Ritalin. My heart sank and I was so upset to learn all that after being told a lie by his doctor, who said there were no side effects and no down side to Ritalin.

I just informed Adam's school this morning that he will no longer be taking meds. They looked at me like I was a complete ass, but my husband and I don't care what they want. We are refusing to medicate Adam. We love him way too much to lose him just to make strangers happy. They were never happy anyhow, always wanting more drugs. His school has no knowledge of ADHD at all. If they did they would work with me, but they will not work with me at all.

When we followed up with Adam's mother two months after she wrote the account above, she remained steadfast in her resolve not the give her son any drugs for ADHD. Curious, we asked how Adam was being treated at school. She reported that his principal and teachers talk about how badly he is doing right in front of him, yet will not give him any extra academic help or intervene if another student acts out against him, among other things. In short, they are punishing Adam and his family and seem intent on doing so until medication is resumed. This is flagrant child abuse, and it is not unusual; we hear similar stories from parent after parent whose children have been victimized by their schools. Fortunately, Adam's family will be moving soon and have heard that the schools in their new town are a lot better. Our fond hope is that this proves to be true.

NO TOLERANCE FOR NORMAL

What could Adam have done to deserve such terrible treatment? Is he a wild, uncontrollable child who is a threat to himself and everybody around him? No. He was targeted simply because he could not sit still long enough to satisfy his school, had too short an attention span for them, and sometimes made noises in class. Like Matt, Stephanie, and millions of others, he committed the sin of acting like a normal child in an environment that only wanted easy to manage, compliant kids.

Francis Fukuyama pegged a significant part of what is going on in his book, *Our Posthuman Future*, when he said, "Ritalin has come to play the role of an overt instrument of social control." What is being controlled is not any kind of aberrant or particularly threatening behavior, but that of normal children who just happen to act in ways that inconvenience adults. The goal of managing normal, even if annoying or inconvenient, childhood behaviors cannot be admitted, of course, because few people would tolerate the use of drugs in pursuit of it. Instead, we hear stories of a burgeoning disease that must be combated. Drugs are much more acceptable in the treatment of disease. But that presents a serious problem.

Though the well-funded search goes on and on for evidence that ADHD is a real condition with a biological basis, none exists. In November of 1998 the National Institutes of Health held a Consensus Conference on ADHD. In the statement released at its conclusion, after hearing from a wide-ranging panel of experts (despite almost all of them being pro ADHD and pro drug), they said, "...we do not have an independent, valid test for ADHD, and there is no data to indicate that ADHD is due to a brain malfunction." These facts have not changed in the time since.

If ADHD is not a brain malfunction then what is it? Again, Francis Fukuyama provides an excellent explanation, "...ADHD isn't a disease at all but rather just the tail of the bell curve describing the distribution of perfectly normal behavior. Young human beings, and particularly young boys, were not designed by evolution to sit around at a desk for hours at a time paying attention to a teacher, but rather to run and play and do other physically active things. The fact that we increasingly demand they sit still in classrooms, or that parents and teachers have less time to spend with them on interesting tasks, is what creates the impression that there is a growing disease."

To further illustrate how labeling a child with a false disease can lead to problems much worse than the original school-based complaints, here is another recent case. Again, the names have been changed, but a mother is telling the story in her own words.

ANGER RISING

Well, the way this all started with my son was in first grade. His teacher had a couple of conferences with me about Chris getting up out of his seat during lessons. If he felt he needed help with something he would go to the teacher or the teacher's helpers (other parents) and tap them on the shoulder and say he didn't understand what he was supposed to be doing. The teacher, the school counselor, and the school psychologist asked to test him to see if he was either too slow for the class or he was bored because the class was too easy. Naturally I agreed. The testing results were split. There were words and meanings he knew that in first grade he should not have known yet, but in math he knew very little. The school psychologist told me he was an average child and that she would like to write up a report from her, his teacher, and the counselor and have me take it to his doctor and have him tested for ADHD, that maybe being put on meds would help him. Never having dealt with this and trusting the school, I agreed.

I took the report and my son to his doctor. He looked it over and asked me if anyone in our family was ADHD. I told him a nephew was. Dr. M wrote my son a prescription for 5 mg of Ritalin. Chris was on and off the meds for the next two years. Then, when he started fourth grade Dr. M. upped the dosage to 10 mg twice a day. After about 4 – 5 months his teacher noticed he was not totally focusing at school and was getting some attitude toward her. So I took him back to Dr. M. and told him what was happening at school. He upped the dosage to 20mg.

This is when I really started to see Chris's anger. His sisters would say something to him (not trying to be mean) and he would fly off the handle, grab them by the ankle, and twist as hard as he could. His dad caught him trying to stab his sister. He punched me in the face.

As the days went on his anger got worse toward his sisters. He would stomp into his room saying how he wished he never was born, that he hated his life. Then, about a week before Christmas

I was sitting at the computer and my son was having a typical day. He came in the computer room and asked if I wanted to see a picture he drew. I said sure. He sat the picture next to me and left the room. I looked at it and saw a picture of him now at age nine and him as an adult. The adult Chris was stabbing the 9-year-old Chris in the head with a big knife and blood was everywhere. The adult Chris had the word "murderer" written across the top of him. I asked my son why he drew that and he said because he can't do nothing right. So I called his doctor and Dr. M. said his anger had nothing to do with the Ritalin. [12] Chris had a deeper psychosis and needed to see a psychologist. He gave me the name of a local psychologist. I never called them because I took Chris off the Ritalin and saw a major difference in attitude.

When school started back after vacation I told my son not to tell his teacher he wasn't taking the Ritalin. His teacher didn't say anything to me or him about anything for almost a week. Then she asked Chris and he told her he wasn't taking the med. She made him feel bad so I wrote her a two page note about why he wasn't taking the Ritalin, the anger, and why keeping him still in school wasn't as important as the safety of my kids. She called me a couple of times at home to let me know Chris was being disruptive and not focusing. I had a meeting with the school counselor and told her under no circumstance was Chris going back on Ritalin. He had been suicidal on it, angry, not sleeping at night, and was never hungry. He went from a size 10 regular jean and lost so much weight you could count his ribs in a size 7 slim jeans. I told the counselor I would work with the teacher to find other solutions.

His teacher started to do her own research on ADHD and Ritalin. She called me last week and we had a long talk. She told me that with what she found out she would never tell a parent to put their child on Ritalin, although she did suggest Adderall. I told her no to Adderall and she dropped the subject and told me that Chris isn't disruptive in class, he just doesn't get the work finished in time.

It is interesting to see at the end of the story that the teacher has educated herself enough to know better than to tell a parent to put a child on Ritalin, but then she goes right ahead and suggests Adderall, an amphetamine that is just as bad. Note, too, that Chris was not even disruptive in class, yet the teacher wanted to continue drugging this poor child, after knowing all that he had been through, just so he could get his work done on time.

Is this what it has come to, the point where our children can be diagnosed and drugged for even small deviations from expectations, expectations that are wrong-headed to begin with? Yes, we have sunk that low, and the crisis is worsening.

A WIDENING PLAGUE

With the successful spread of the ADHD plague serving as a template, we now see diagnoses like anxiety, depression, bipolar, obsessive compulsive, and many others rampaging through the child population. We certainly do not claim that children have no real problems or never exhibit disturbing behaviors. Plenty of them do, but these are almost always in response to adverse situations in their environments, which are controlled by adults, and not dysfunctions in their brains, which have become the popular scapegoats. Troubled kids need real help, not chemical restraints administered by adults who refuse to address the true issues. When a child feels sad, distressed, or worried, when a child's moods go up and down or she acts out with violence, sex, or drugs, there is surely something wrong that needs to be fixed, maybe something very wrong—but it's not in their brains, it's in how we, the adults who are responsible for them, are conducting ourselves.

Today we have reached the sad state where, according to a 2002 study conducted by Yale University, 9 of 10 children who visit a child psychiatrist are given a prescription for a psychotropic drug. [13] In this sad state the discipline of psychiatry serves as the administering arm of pharmaceutical companies who collude with them to invent diseases for profit, with no consideration given to the real needs of children, their futures, or their very lives. We are told this is being done in the best interest of suffering children, a lie that goes beyond mere hypocrisy. C.S. Lewis provided an apt description of this state of affairs when he wrote, "There is no tyranny so great as that which is practiced for the victim."

THE REAL VILLIANS

For most of us parents it isn't the iconic dealer down by the corner we need to fear when it comes to drugs. It is the schools that post signs saying they are "drug free zones," the health care professionals who make livings by tarring kids with bogus labels, the insurance companies who view drug treatments as more cost-effective, the pharmaceutical companies who make billions by making poisons appear as safe, and lots more beneficial, than Flintstone vitamins. The most effective drug pushers are the legal ones.

Chapter Two

MAKING MONKEYS

We're making great progress, but we're headed in the wrong direction.

- Ogden Nash

Millions of people in New Delhi, India, and the surrounding area were swept up in a panic during the spring of 2001. What were they afraid of? A marauding half-man, half-beast creature dubbed the "Monkey Man," a thing so fearsome that the police were flooded with complaints that the creature was terrorizing citizens at night and attacking them with its iron claws. There were pictures in the newspapers of people showing off the wounds they claimed were inflicted by him. Such were his powers reputed to be that some even believed the Monkey Man a super-powered robot being directed by remote control, or maybe even an extra-terrestrial sent here to wreak havoc on any human unfortunate enough to cross its path.

Two men seeking an escape from the Monkey Man climbed to the roofs of buildings and jumped to their deaths. A pregnant woman sleeping on the terrace of her apartment was awakened one night by her neighbor's shouts of "The monkey has come!" In the effort to escape him she fell down a flight of stairs and died. And not everybody had a chance to flee; one woman simply fainted at what she thought was the sight of the Monkey Man on her terrace. Thankfully, she later woke to find him gone and herself unharmed. Many parents sent their children away to live with relatives and friends in safe locations, wanting to keep their children out of danger until this roof-hopping terror was captured. Others refused to leave their home for work. What job is worth the risk of being attacked when you venture outside just to get to it?

At the height of the panic 3,000 police officers were deployed to find and apprehend the monster. By then they had received hundreds of complaints from people who had sighted the monster or claimed to have been bitten or clawed by him. Roving bands of vigilantes patrolled the streets at night, firing guns into the air and feeding the panic even more. Though none of them ever found the Monkey Man, they did attack a few people they mistook for him, including a 4-foot-tall Hindu mystic who was discovered performing rituals in the woods.

Newspapers and television broadcasts followed the search and regularly reported the Monkey Man's attacks, compounding the fears of a frightened populace by continuing to feature those who claimed the horrible beast had inflicted harm on them. Despite the addition of a 50,000 rupee reward ($1,067) to the ongoing efforts to round him up, the Monkey Man was never captured, not by the vigilantes or the official forces of justice. A couple months after the original sightings Indian police concluded that the Monkey Man did not exist and that the panic was a product of mass hysteria. The *Times* of India quoted police sources as saying the creature was a "Mere figment of the imagination of emotionally weak people." Despite numerous reports of physical injury and psychological trauma, an expert report stated "...no one had actually seen it."

THE MAKING OF MONKEYS

To view the Monkey Man panic as simply an example of what happens when fear grips the minds of ignorant people who possess nowhere near the wisdom and clear judgment of those of us in the United States, and foolishly stoke the fires by immediately spreading their irrational visions to others, would be easy. It would also be dead wrong. For we are swept up in our own hoax, one that has lasted many years and becomes steadily worse as trusted health and educational professionals, the media, pharmaceutical companies, insurance companies, and frightened parents fuel it. Compared with what we are engaged in, the Monkey Man scare was a little hiccup of a fright that was soon squelched by reason. If only we were so rational.

Imagine coming across a story about a country where six million children are being drugged with powerful substances to control unwanted behaviors, such as fidgeting, daydreaming, fooling around in class, not paying close enough attention, failing to complete work quickly enough, and acting without sufficient impulse control or self regulation. Imagine a country where the children's very teachers function as front line troops who mark the monkeys in need of chemical correction, with school psychologists, counselors, social workers, and administrators serving as support forces that help broaden the territory under control. Imagine a place where physicians become functionaries who dutifully shock the monkeys' systems with drugs to pacify them.

THE BIG CON

And what of the parents in this place? Why do they allow this massive assault on their children? For some, a drug is a welcome alternative to investing the effort necessary to provide competent parenting. For the most part, though, parents want the best for their children and do not realize how badly they are being led astray.

Parents are told that their targeted children are victims of an unseen force that causes them to act inappropriately. If it is not treated quickly a lifetime of failure, frustration, underachievement, and worse await them. After being duly frightened, parents are given the "good news" that there are safe, mild substances that can tame the beast wreaking havoc in their children's brains. The inference for parents is made very clear—to deny their children these life rafts is akin to leaving them adrift in dangerous waters. What mom or dad could possibly be so irresponsible?

Parents who resist are generously urged to try saving their children on a trial basis; won't they give at least that much a shake? If the magic elixir works, then we have proof that the child really was afflicted. If not, fine, no harm in trying to save a life, right? Of course, when a child is being given a test run of the magic elixir glowing reports come from those who sell it, about how much happier their serum of choice made the child - and will save him from becoming an outcast monkey permanently. Now he fits in and his future is so much brighter. Thank god the monkey mongers took the time to intervene.

What parents are not told is that once they start going along with the monkey-making process turning back is frowned upon. And if the carrot no longer works, the stick is brought out. Michael and Jill Carroll learned this harsh lesson the hard way, when they were threatened with the loss of their children. Their son, Kyle, entered kindergarten as an energetic, curious, sometimes goofy, exuberant five-year-old; a normal boy. His teacher, worried that he wouldn't be able to sit still enough for first grade, recommended that he be evaluated for ADHD. Kyle's parents followed the recommendation and soon he was on Ritalin. The early months of first grade went okay on the drug, but things began to go downhill in the spring term.

Kyle began having trouble sleeping at night, often coming home completely exhausted from school. His appetite deteriorated and he began complaining of pains in his legs he called the "wigglies." As his father told *Redbook* magazine in October of 2001, "One of the scariest things about this was watching his personality change. [1] You could see it in his eyes. There was an absence of anything going on." When the final report card of the year arrived and the grades were poor, it was the last straw, Kyle's parents took him off Ritalin. He took remedial classes over the summer and had no problems in school. "He was back to normal, doing the things kids do instead of being so lethargic," his father reports.

When second grade began Michael and Jill decided to try him without the Ritalin. On the second day the school nurse called to find out why he wasn't being given the drug. Mr. Carroll detailed the problems they saw as a result of Ritalin and explained their rationale in stopping it. Soon after this conversation the school called the Albany County Department of Social Services and claimed that the decision to discontinue the Ritalin endangered Kyle's ability to function at school. A social worker came to the Carroll's home and informed them that they could be charged with medical neglect if they did not give Kyle Ritalin. In the same *Redbook* article, Michael Carroll said, "I was scared I was going to lose custody of my son and possibly my other children too."

That October, in a meeting with a school guidance counselor and psychologist, the Carrolls were told that not giving Kyle Ritalin was like withholding insulin from a diabetic. On every page of his IEP (Individualized Educational Plan) was the phrase, "Medication is important for educational success." The Carrolls yielded to the accumulating pressure and resumed medication, which continued until the following year when their pediatrician agreed to stop prescribing it due to the parents' continuing alarm over the harm Ritalin did to their son.

Are schools correct when they assert drugs like Ritalin are necessary for school success? No. As James Swanson, a professor of pediatrics, found in a 1993 review of the research, Ritalin results in no long-term improvements in academic functioning. Not only that, this same Dr. Swanson, in answer to a question on making the ADHD diagnosis that was posed to him at the March 7, 1998 meeting of the American Society of Adolescent Psychiatry, replied, "I would like to have an objective diagnosis for the disorder (ADHD). Right now psychiatric diagnosis is completely subjective...We would like to have biological tests, a dream of psychiatry for many years."

For children like Kyle who are targeted by their schools and identified as monkeys in a diagnostic frenzy for chemical means of restraint, their interests and very health are sacrificed solely to make them easier to manage in school. As Jill Carroll said in the February, 2001, issue of *Reason* magazine, "Ritalin solved the problem for the school, but the side effects were too much."

There is nothing so monstrous about normal childhood behavior that it warrants the millions of seek-and-destroy missions that have been launched against it, with the label of ADHD used in the attempt to provide a legitimate cover. The school side of the story always focuses on how disruptive a few misbehaving children can be to a classroom, about how high student/teacher ratios makes it necessary to quiet the uncooperative minority. But latching on to drugs because they are perceived to make classroom management easier is not the answer.

The real horror is that adults are willing to mount such a horrendous assault on childhood itself. Diane McGuinness, the author of *When Children Don't Learn* and a psychologist who did her own review of the research literature said, "Methodologically rigorous research indicates that attention deficit disorder and hyperactivity as syndromes simply do not exist. We have invented a disease, given it a medical solution, and now must disown it. The major question is how we go about destroying the monster we have created."

In India the Monkey Man panic ended when it was shown to be false. Here in the United States, the complete absence of any evidence our own Monkey Man exists, in the form of ADHD, only makes those who believe in it more determined to find "proof," or, at least, things that can be dressed up to look like proof.

In India, the feared and hunted Monkey Man was not seen as "one of us." It was an outside force that needed to be combated in order to keep the children safe, an admirable motive even though the specter was nonexistent. Here in the United States we have been conned into believing that the evil force resides in our own children, a Monkey Man of the brain that takes the form of attention deficit hyperactivity disorder, and we hunt for those kids so infected with the monstrosity. There is one thing the Monkey Man hoax in India and the ADHD hoax in America share in common. They have each been viewed exactly the same number of times — never.

In India a handful of people were mistakenly attacked in the belief that they were the Monkey Man. After the episode ended it is reasonable to assume the attacks did, too. Here in America innocent children are stuck with labels that can stigmatize and harm them for life. They have been told that any conflicts they have with adult authorities are evidence of misfiring brains, just as any scratch or gouge could be used to prove there was a Monkey Man afoot, and then forced to take powerful, addictive drugs that can permanently damage them. Worse yet, these children are taught to continue inflicting harm on themselves by being convinced they have a lifetime handicapping condition and may never be "right." Not only have they been identified as monkeys by adults, they are now taught to identify themselves as such.

In both India and the United States, the respective fears we have been discussing did have some factual basis in the beginning, before they took off into the nether regions. In New Delhi there had long been a problem with monkeys roaming the city who had been known to pounce on people, so the prospect of some kind of super-charged monkey going on the offensive against citizens is not as far fetched as it first appears. Similarly, children have always acted in ways that bug adults, particularly in school settings where institutional requirements so often go against the grain of their evolving selves.

A SHOCK TO THE SYSTEM

Both authors first became aware of the growing ADHD plague when their sons were targeted for the diagnosis. Though the incidents were almost 30 years apart (Fred's son in 1971 and

Craig's son in 2000) they are very similar in the respective schools' attempts to make monkeys of normal boys.

A NEUROLOGIST'S NIGHTMARE

The proudest day of my life (senior author Fred Baughman) was the day I was accepted to medical school at New York University. After graduating I went on to specialize in neurology, which I practiced in Grand Rapids, Michigan, then San Diego, California. In addition to a busy private practice of adult and child neurology, I maintained an active presence in neurological research, where I discovered and verified several neurological and genetic diseases.

During the 60s and 70s I became concerned with the increasing numbers of psychiatric and learning disorders children were being diagnosed with. None of these were ever verified with real evidence or legitimate research, yet they were described as existing in the same sense as the physical diseases I saw daily, in my practice.

The issue hit home in 1971 when a teacher and school principal claimed our 7-year-old son, Duane, suffered from "hyperactive child syndrome," a label that was a precursor to what we know as attention deficit/hyperactivity disorder today, and needed to be put on Ritalin. Duane's response was to state plainly, "I'm not a 'mental,' I don't need that stuff." If not "mental," then what? Duane was simply a bright, energetic child who clashed with the standards of his school, for which he was rewarded with the school's opinion that he suffered from an unproven neurological disease.

Both I and my wife, Annette, a devoted and no-nonsense mother who would have none of the label the school wanted to affix to her son, knew there was nothing wrong with Duane. A wonderful 2nd grade teacher volunteered to take Duane in her class the following year and was able to keep his energies directed appropriately and teach him. No more mention was made of

Duane suffering from any kind of disorder or needing medication. Today, Duane operates his own business and does, I might add, exceedingly well at it, no thanks to psychiatry or Ritalin. The energy, drive, and intelligence he showed as a child serve him very well in a field where these qualities are valued and rewarded. Sadly, far too many of the Duanes of today are judged to be defective by their schools because they are not easy enough to manage and do not fit compliantly into adult-managed educational environments, with the result being diagnoses and drugs. We are only beginning to get an inkling of what we as a society and, more importantly, the mislabeled children themselves, have lost out on as a result.

If the condition Duane's school claimed he had were real, then no amount of good teaching would have cured it. You can't cure a broken leg with good teaching—real medical intervention is called for. That none was needed is evidence that there was nothing wrong with him to begin with.

Back when Duane's school sought to have him diagnosed and drugged there were "only" 150,000-200,000 American children labeled with the early versions of ADHD. The numbers increased steadily throughout the 70s, rose at a more rapid pace during the 80s, and exploded in the 90s.

Early in the 80s growing numbers of children were referred to me by schools and family physicians for confirmation of their diagnoses of what was now called attention deficit disorder (ADD). I went through the medical literature on it and could find no evidence that it was a legitimate diagnosis. More importantly, the children referred to me whose schools were convinced suffered from brain abnormalities were normal; I could find nothing wrong with them. Imagine my shock, when after thoroughly examining a child and finding him to be perfectly okay, I would be contacted by school personnel who insisted that I either make the ADD diagnosis and write a prescription for Ritalin or the school would see to it that the family found another physician who would.

I refused to bow to the pressure. How in the world could people with no medical training override my judgment (after all, I am the neurologist here)? How could a teacher, school psychologist, principal, social worker, or counselor tell me, a physician whose area of expertise was the human brain, that a child suffered from a brain disease, especially one for which there is no evidence? I did everything I could to keep children I saw from being diagnosed and given dangerous drugs that had no business in a child's body or brain, but the stampede to tag kids with ADHD and medicate them into compliance was beyond my powers alone to stem. For every normal child I was able to steer away from the fraudulent diagnosis and drugs thousands more became some other doctor's patients.

During the 90s I was horrified to see the stampede turn into a plague—a nationwide and worldwide plague. In 1987, when the current ADHD formulation began being used, there were 500,000 children being treated with stimulants, then 1,000,000 by 1990, and up to 6 million children diagnosed with ADHD by the end of the decade. Not only was there still no proof that ADHD existed or any kind of objective test for it, which went against everything in my medical and scientific training and experience, but the drugs being forced on children had a long and well-documented history of being dangerous, risky substances that came with a long list of unpleasant side effects, including addiction and death.

All of the stimulants prescribed for ADHD are classified as Schedule II drugs by the Drug Enforcement Agency (DEA), a classification reserved for the most dangerous and addictive drugs that can be legally prescribed. As mentioned above, Ritalin, the most popular ADHD drug in the past and still the best known, is very similar to amphetamines and cocaine. During the 90s another ADHD drug was introduced that overtook Ritalin as the most commonly prescribed by the year 2000, Adderall, a mixture of amphetamine salts. This was not a new drug specifically developed for children, it has been around for years. Adderall used to be called Obetrol and was prescribed mainly to women who wanted to lose weight. It was taken off the market in 1981 because so many women had become addicted to it, which should come as no surprise considering the long and well-documented history of amphetamine abuse. A few years ago I read that one of the best known ADHD researchers, Peter S. Jensen [2] of Columbia University, had refused Ritalin and Adderall treatment of his own child when he was diagnosed with ADHD. I suspect Jensen did so because he knows more about the proven dangers of these drugs than most parents, though this has not stopped him from advocating for court orders to treat children with the same drugs if their parents refuse to comply.

What was horrifying to me and to physicians of conscience across the country is that Obertol was repackaged, given a new name, and, after an intense, expensive, and successful promotional campaign, became the drug of choice for children for many thousands of physicians, despite its history. Not only was I shocked by the lack of ethics seen in a pharmaceutical company's efforts to have children given a drug that had already been clearly established as a danger to them, I was also amazed that so many of my fellow physicians were either unaware or unconcerned over the dangers Adderall and similar drugs posed to children. In 1996 Gene Haslip of the DEA addressed this problem in his concluding statement at the end of a conference on stimulant use in the treatment of ADHD. The drug specifically referred to below is Ritalin, but the same applies to Adderall and each of the stimulants children are forced to take for ADHD.

> *Parents need to understand that we are talking about very potent, addictive and abusable substances...Regretably, much of the literature and promotion of the drug in recent years has ignored or understated the potency and abuse potential of methylphenidate and Ritalin. This appears to have misled many physicians into prescribing the drug as a quick-fix for learning and behavior problems.*

Indeed, the ADHD drugs are quick fixes, as the majority of children who take them become subdued, over-focused, and compliant soon after taking them. [3] Between 1990 and Gene Haslip's 1996 statement, Ritalin prescriptions increased 500%; amphetamine (drugs like Dexedrine and Adderall) prescriptions for ADHD increased by 400%; 7-10% of boys in school were estimated to be on these drugs, along with a rising percentage of girls. In some districts 15-20% of the children were being diagnosed and drugged for ADHD. Much to my distress, the pharmaceutical companies were raking in fortunes from selling these drugs, with profits alone rising to around $500 million a year. As drug profits skyrocketed, so also did injuries and deaths suffered from abusing these drugs. There was a 1000% increase in these reported for Ritalin alone in children aged 10 to 14. According to Mr. Haslip, "This now equals or exceeds reports for the same age group involving cocaine."

As a physician and father, I became increasingly disturbed as the numbers of children labeled ADHD skyrocketed. To be diagnosed as ADHD all a child has to do is be observed committing sins like fidgeting, talking out of turn, getting out of her chair, playing too loudly, not completing assignments, and pretty much anything that might irritate a teacher. I witnessed childhood itself being termed a disease (see Chapter 5 for an analysis of the diagnostic criteria).

ADHD "experts" emerged during the 80s and 90s who made their livings advocating the targeting of children who annoyed adults. Using scientific sounding language, with no actual scientific evidence to back up their opinions, they provided justifications for the wholesale drugging of noncompliant children. Perhaps the best known, and among the most dangerous, of these experts is Russell Barkley, who said in 1991, "Although inattention, overactivity, and poor impulse control are the most common symptoms cited by others as primary in hyperactive children, my own work with these children suggests that noncompliance is also a primary problem." He goes on to say, "...there is, in fact, something 'wrong' with these children." What Barkley and others of his ilk did, and continue to do, is provide a legitimate sounding excuse for making normal aspects of childhood itself a disease and excuse the forcible administration of dangerous drugs. In short, I witnessed the growth of a new class of health care professionals who advocated child abuse under the guise of "treatment."

The Barkleys of the world encouraged teachers, psychologists, physicians, and parents to see the problem as only residing within the malfunctioning brain of the child, without giving nearly enough attention to their family situations, lack of fit with schools, and any number of other factors, like human nature itself, that cause children to come into conflict with adults. The more you listen to them the more you realize that noncompliance is the core problem they seek to extinguish. This is also where the entire diagnosis falls apart—noncompliance is not a medical condition.

As a neurologist who saw thousands of children during my 35 years of practice I knew how much variation there was in learning styles, aptitudes, rates of development, temperament, personality, and a host of other factors in children, some of whom developed at a faster pace than others, some who developed slower. As children grew and, hopefully, with adult support, they learned how to direct and control themselves and find the ways of interacting with their environments that worked best, given each individual child's unique blend of attributes. I also knew how much children's school performance could be affected by what was going on at a home, such as parents splitting up and other forms of family turmoil—but a divorce does not cause disease. Yet, now children by the hundreds of thousands were being diagnosed with an unproven disease, based on criteria so broad and subjective almost any child could be tagged with ADHD, given dangerous, addictive drugs, while all factors relating to their uniqueness as individuals or the environments they came from were ignored. Never in my medical experience had I seen anything like this happen.

As a researcher who has discovered and verified real diseases, I am familiar with the rigorous scientific standards that have to be met before claiming that a new, unique, disease exists. Now, teachers were making ADHD diagnoses as though they had been deputized and vested with some special power that overcame their lack of medical training, expertise, or experience. They were able to do so because the diagnostic criteria for ADHD and all its predecessors were so subjective and broad that anybody could find a way to diagnose any child they wanted to. All a child had to do was demonstrate a few of the common childhood characteristics listed from a menu of them, things like not paying enough attention to details, making careless mistakes in homework, not listening, not maintaining attention, losing things, becoming distracted, being forgetful or fidgety, getting out of a chair, moving when being seated is called for, talking too much, being impulsive, interrupting, blurting out answers, and committing the sin of being impatient while awaiting a turn at something. Just the observance of a few of these is enough for a medical diagnosis and the administration of stimulants. I found stimulant treatment particularly senseless because these are the very kinds of drugs that can cause many of the problems listed above. The response to that, of course, is to pile on more diagnoses and add ever more powerful drugs to a child's system, which is the point we have reached today.

NO DIFFERENCE ALLOWED

My own (co-author Craig Hovey) experience with ADHD began when a 6th grade teacher and school psychologist told me my son, Max, had it. They presented it as a real disease, like diabetes, a condition that would result in a lifetime of misery and failure for him if it was not properly diagnosed and treated with medication, the medication being the equivalent of glasses to help a near-sighted person or insulin for a diabetic.

This was not the first time educators had informed me that my son's brain was malfunctioning. They did that during the first year he attended elementary school in the suburban district we moved to shortly before he began 4th grade. Through 3rd grade Max attended elementary school in a poorly performing urban school district and, like me at that age, he was a behind most other children in the development of his reading skills. Making matters worse was the city district using whole language to teach reading at the time, an approach that has proven to be a miserable failure. It was no surprise when the academically superior suburban school came to my wife and me with concerns over Max's performance.

We explained all of the above factors to them, along with our observation that he was an athletic, social kid whose learning style was an active rather than passive one. They listened politely, nodded, smiled as us, and ignored every word we spoke. When the school psychologist, counselor, and a teacher or two expressed the opinion that Max was learning disabled we knew better than to swallow it. The problem was, however, that school then was a difficult and frustrating experience for him. The smaller class size of a special education class would mean more attention and less damage to his self-esteem, or so we thought. We went for it.

At the first annual meeting to review his progress, a statement on one of his evaluation forms came to light that shocked us. It read, "age appropriate when on medication." Max was on no medication and not a single person at his school had said a word to us about his having any kind of condition that required it, yet. Was it an error? I doubt it. Max's school had pegged him for ADHD and needing medication well before they said anything to us. They had already been successful in targeting hundreds, or probably thousands, of other kids for the ADHD diagnosis and drugs, and Max was just one more, with one more set of parents who could be bullied and manipulated into going along with them.

It has been our good fortune to have a wonderful pediatrician. After the teacher and school psychologist informed me Max had ADHD, I brought him to her and she dismissed the notion as "ridiculous." It was also my good fortune at the time to have a colleague at the college I taught at who is a neurobiologist and familiar with the research on ADHD. He made it clear that there is no evidence that ADHD exists and that the brains of children diagnosed with it are no different than other children's (that is, before stimulants are introduced), despite claims to the contrary that have never been backed up with any real evidence.

In addition to Max being behind grade level and having an active learning style there is another factor I am certain played a role. Max is a mixed child (one black and one white parent). It is interesting to note that black males are approximately three times more likely than white males to wind up in special education classes. Now, when a student is labeled learning disabled the assumption is that it is the result of a central nervous malfunction, which means an abnormality or disease of the brain. Since there is no difference in the brains of black versus white people, why are black males so much more likely to be judged to have a malfunctioning brain? It is no longer acceptable to state prejudice outright; doing so under cover of an official label (albeit one with no scientific basis) can be gotten away with, however. Schools seem to tolerate children who are members of minority groups okay if they "behave" appropriately, which means acting like nice middle class white kids, but if they deviate from the norms they are targeted to a greater degree than a similar acting white child. So much for the wonders of diversity.

We also found, as have so many of the parents I have spoken to in researching this book, that once a child is labeled as ADHD, learning disabled, or a problem in any way, it follows them right through a school system. For example, we took Max out of special education at the end of 7th grade because the services provided were poor, damaging to his self-esteem and, since he was not learning disabled to begin with, unnecessary. Unfortunately, he had already been tagged as a problem, even though his behavior was never particularly bad for a kid his age, and the tag stuck, even when he went on to high school.

Two weeks into his freshman year a teacher took him out into the hall and informed him that his other teachers were talking about him because he was unfocussed and disruptive in class and badly behaved in the hallways outside of them. Her message to him was clear: we all know you are a problem, we communicate with each other about it, and you better be extra careful because we are on alert for the next time you mess up. Fortunately, my wife had just contacted Max's teachers a couple days earlier (the teacher who targeted him co-taught a course and her colleague was among them) and heard from every one of them that he was doing well in his classes and was not having any problems at all. I looked into it further and discovered there really were no alarms over him being sounded and the teachers were not having discussion sessions about how to deal with this huge threat of a mixed-race freshman. The teacher, acting on her own, had taken it on herself to single him out. The lesson here is that it does not take a well-organized conspiracy of educators to damage your child. A few can be plenty.

The point I'm making to parents is that once you allow your child to be identified as a problem or having a problem of any kind, there is a real danger of the ante being continually upped with discoveries of new, even worse, problems, and labels that stick, and stick some more.

As parents, we know our children better than the schools do. It is very rare to speak with a parent whose child is diagnosed as ADHD where the initial suggestion of it and push for diagnosis did not come from a school. As parents, it is time we stood up to schools that have become more and more intolerant of children over the years. Today, a child who deviates from the norms of placid adults in any way is in danger of being targeted by his or her school, and once that bull's eye is drawn on them it probably will not be erased, and if the child has been taught to label herself, the condition, sadly, can become permanent, a permanent hurt.

As I write Max is doing great and has experienced the good fortune of finding success outside of school. He has developed a passion for hockey and is pursuing it with a discipline, drive, intelligence, and focus that I doubt any of the educators so bent on branding him as disabled have ever come close to exhibiting.

Maybe they need some kind of special medication that enhances ambition and the energy to fulfill it. Or maybe they could try to overcome their disabilities and learn from Max's example.

TREATING NORMAL BEHAVIOR
AS ABNORMAL

William Carey, M.D., a highly respected pediatrician, professor, and researcher with many years of experience, in his 1998 testimony before the National Institutes of Health, said, "What is now most often described as ADHD in the United States appears to be a set of normal behavior variations that sometimes lead to dysfunction through dissonant environmental interactions. This discrepancy leaves the validity of the construct in doubt." [4]

In short, the things that bother adults about how children act, particularly in school, have been grouped together in a set of undesirable behaviors whose existence is claimed to be the result of an abnormality that only resides in the child, with the adults involved sharing little of the responsibility when there is a lack of fit between a child and the adult-controlled environment he lives in.

There is no more correlation between what used to be regarded as normal childhood behaviors and ADHD than there is between a scratch on the back and a marauding Monkey Man. When asked by a parent, at a Drug Enforcement Agency conference on the use of stimulant treatment for ADHD in 1996, if there was any evidence to back up the existence of ADHD, Dr. Lawrence Diller (author of *Running on Ritalin* and *Should I Medicate My Child?*) responded, "The reason why you have been unable to obtain any articles or studies presenting clear and confirming evidence of a physical or chemical abnormality associated with ADHD is that there is none." The proponents of ADHD remain convinced that evidence will eventually be found, if only they look long enough for this holy grail ("That monkey's got to be around here somewhere").

The shame of it is that once children are labeled with ADHD they are no longer treated as normal. Once psychotropic drugs like Ritalin begin coursing through their brains and bodies they become, for the first time, physically, neurologically, and biologically abnormal. And the process does not stop here, for, once a child is seen as abnormal, the door opens wide for a host of other labels and drugs, especially if the child does not respond as hoped to the initial drugging. A monkey has been made.

Below is the story of Paul Johnston, which is a telling example of just how horrifying things can get.

THE BOY WHO WAS MISTAKEN FOR A MONKEY

Soon after Paul Johnston began kindergarten his mother, Joy, was called in for a meeting with the teacher. This teacher took it on herself to inform Joy that Paul was an ADHD child, a boy who suffered from a brain disorder just like those seen in children whose mothers drank alcohol during pregnancy (Joy had not). What evidence did the teacher have? She claimed that Paul, age 5, was disrupting the class by not waiting his turn to answer questions, was fidgety, and would not do his work with the rest of the children. Because she had received some training in how to identify ADHD children she felt she understood the problem. Paul's teacher went on to tell Joy that nearly 30% of all children, mainly boys, suffered from ADHD. According to Joy, Paul's kindergarten class contained 21 children; at least 5 of the 10 boys in it had already been identified as ADHD and were taking Ritalin. The teacher referred Joy to the same doctor who had written prescriptions for the other boys.

Joy and her husband viewed Paul as a normal boy and held off on making an appointment, deciding that they would work with him on following rules, not making too much noise, etc. They thought things were going okay, until the school principal called a couple weeks later. He was upset about Paul's behavior and said the boy was going to be suspended if something wasn't done to get him under control. At home Paul was a normal 5 year-old. What could be so different at school? When Joy met with the principal and teacher the following week and questioned them on their continued insistence that he was an ADHD child with serious behavior problems, they responded by informing her that Child Protective Services would be called in for medical neglect if she continued to ignore the problem. Joy felt she didn't have a choice, so she took Paul to that doctor Paul's teacher recommended and he was put on Ritalin. Beyond the behaviors the teacher had originally spoken of, none too unusual for a boy in kindergarten, Paul hadn't started committing any additional sins. It seems that Joy's questioning the school's judgment and wanting more details only served to aggravate them and increase their determination to get him medicated.

In his office, the doctor seemed more interested in the note Paul's teacher had given Joy to bring along than in Paul himself. He claimed the Ritalin he prescribed would help Paul control his behavior and become better able to concentrate on his school-work. Over the next several weeks Paul's teacher claimed to see improvements in how he functioned and said the medication was working. Joy, however, was becoming increasingly concerned because Paul was becoming moody, had trouble sleeping, and was not eating much. Over the summer, Paul became aggressive and short-tempered. When informed of this, their doctor increased the Ritalin dosage, despite the fact that aggression, lack of appetite, and trouble sleeping are all well-known side effects of Ritalin, which, remember, is a powerful stimulant, not "mild" as it is usually described to parents. Yet, instead of backing off on the medication, Paul's doctor upped it. Is it any surprise that things only got worse from here?

Over the next seven years Paul was put on an ever- stronger mix of medications for the lengthening list of disorders he was diagnosed with, by many different doctors. Dexedrine, another stimulant, was added to the Ritalin, then the Ritalin was stopped and Cylert (a drug already taken off the market in Canada because it can lead to liver failure and death) was added, followed by a switch to Adderall. None of them, or any combination, worked any better. Now Paul's moods were running wild, from hyper to tired, so Tofranil, an antidepressant (a tricyclic antidepressant, kin to desipramine, a drug that has killed a reported eight children and probably many more) was prescribed to accompany the Adderall. [5] [6] [7]

Soon Paul began having terrible headaches and bad dreams to go along with his continued moodiness, aggression, lethargy, and weight loss. Then he began having hallucinations at night, of monsters who chased him and told him to do bad things. Auditory and visual hallucinations are among the dissociative reactions that can be brought on by antidepressants. In *Psychiatric Drugs Explained*, psychiatrist Dr. David Healy states, "The danger of these dissociative experiences lies in the fact that they may be interpreted by either the person taking the antidepressant or others as evidence that the illness is getting worse or that brain damage of some sort has been caused that may be permanent. If misinterpreted, such reactions can lead on to suicide... This risk, and the fact that a drug causing such reactions is most unlikely to cure depression, provide grounds for switching treatment to something else." Paul remained on Tofranil. He tried to kill himself twice. The first time Paul's sister found him in the basement, stabbing himself in the chest with shears. The second occasion came when Paul gulped down a bottle of pills. Lucky for him they were only an antibiotic.

Paul wound up in an institution for severely disturbed and dangerous juveniles. Along the way his original ADHD diagnosis was followed up with those of bi-polar disorder, schizoaffective disorder, and oppositional defiant disorder. In addition to the Tofranil and ADHD medications, Paul was put on Depakote, Wellbutrin, Risperdal, and Seroquel, none of whose effects have been studied in children, nor have they been approved by the FDA for use in children. [8]

Nobody really knows how any of these drugs work, alone or in combination, and for children forced to take them it is the drug itself that becomes their first real abnormality, their first disease.

Paul is out of the institution now, drug-free and being schooled at home, but he did not escape free from damage. A few months after securing his release Joy related that, "The medication damaged my son before I was able to withdraw it from his system. He was left suffering from visual disturbances (like someone who took LSD), Tardive Dyskinesia (involuntary, tic-like, and writhing movements, often permanent—a real brain abnormality/disease usually due to antipsychotic drugs such as the Risperdal, and Seroquel he was on), and PTSD (post traumatic stress disorder— not a physical disease) because of the abuse he suffered from the system. While in the institution he was beaten, burned, tied up in bed sheets with a sock stuffed in his mouth, and medicated with the highest amount of psychiatric drugs they could use without killing him...just to keep him quiet." All of these horrors were suffered by a boy who had nothing wrong with him, a boy whose nightmare began only because he acted his age in kindergarten, in a school unwilling to tolerate that sin.

* * *

As bad as Paul's experiences were, other children are not even that fortunate. In 1991 Cameron Pettus was diagnosed with ADHD and put on desipramine, an anti-depressant sometimes used to treat ADHD. Two years later he died of an allergic reaction to the drug that had destroyed his heart, liver, and lungs. As usual, the diagnostic process got started after a teacher complained that Cameron had trouble sitting still in school. His mother believes the real issues were the stress of she and Cameron's father getting divorced and Cameron having an active learning style. The same has happened to countless children, kids reacting to serious problems in their lives or simply not being the kinds of learners their teachers want to see in front of them. Do these issues matter to school personnel? Not if the child has become an inconvenience to a teacher-turned-diagnostician with a label in mind.

At the time Cameron was prescribed desipramine, six children were already known to have died from the drug, yet the parents were never informed of its dangers. Not only do school personnel routinely push drugs whose dangers they have little knowledge of, many physicians (and child psychiatrists are the worst offenders) do the same. In the March 21, 1999, edition of *The Austin American Statesman*, Cameron's mother said, "If somebody had told me this was a potentially deadly drug, I never would have given it to him." Ever since Cameron's death, desipramine continues to be prescribed for children, and more deaths have followed.

In a May 24, 2002, article for Salon.com, Dr. Lawrence Diller addressed the death of another child from desipramine in 2001 (the story is told in detail here in Chapter Four) stating, "Shaina Dunkle should never have been on this drug." Desipramine had been presented to Shaina's parents as a safe alternative to Ritalin, without that drug's potential for abuse. Like Cameron's parents before them, never were they told of the risks involved, never were they told that at least seven children had already died suddenly from desipramine by the mid-90s. Recall what we said in the first chapter: reported occurrences have been found to be only a small portion of the actual. Who knows for sure how many children have died from desipramine – or will in the future?

A COLLECTIVE MADNESS

In a July, 2001, interview with the *New Jersey Times*, the novelist James Lee Burke said, "The greatest injustices are usually done in a collective way in which no individual becomes responsible." This is precisely what has happened with the plague of psychiatric diagnoses in children. The individuals who participate in the effort to diagnosis and drug ever more millions of children are mostly (with some notable exceptions) decent people with a sense of morality who have convinced themselves, or been convinced, with no real evidence, that what they are doing is right. But what they are doing—feeding psychoactive drugs to children—makes no more sense than burning witches at the stake.

By acting in their own interests, the different parties involved have created a vast market for ADHD and other invented disorders. Schools have always longed for a simple and effective means of dealing with children who do not jibe well with the requirements of the classroom. Drug manufacturers constantly seek to expand their markets and have found a windfall in the ADHD drugs with revenues for these alone hitting $1 billion in 2001. Health care providers have an expanding patient base to draw from as the numbers of ADHD cases continue to rise. Insurance companies, who typically pay a physician for no more than 15 minutes of their time to evaluate a child for ADHD, save money when drugs like Adderall and Ritalin are prescribed instead of delving into a more labor-intensive examination of what the real home or school problems might be.

None of the above parties intentionally harm children, though they consistently deny or ignore the harm their actions cause, yet the sum of their actions add up to child abuse on a massive scale. And what of the parents who go along? For the most part, they are trying to be as responsible as possible. Rarely do they realize how colossally misinformed they have been because they trust that these experts know what they are doing and are acting in the best interest of their children. And though the argument is made that the experts really are doing what they think is best, they should know better and not be so willing to shovel out misinformation or swallow it themselves, especially considering the complete lack of real evidence that ADHD is an actual disease or disorder of any kind.

As Dr. William Carey pointed out during his testimony at the NIH Consensus Conference on ADHD, "The DSM-IV [The American Psychiatric Association's guide to psychiatric diagnoses] does not say so but virtually all articles in the professional journals and textbooks assume that the ADHD behaviors of high activity and low attention span are largely or entirely due to abnormal brain function." For example, the great majority of books, articles, pamphlets, and web sites on ADHD refer to it as the most common neurobehavioral disorder (neuro—a nervous system abnormality) in childhood, despite it never coming close to meeting any scientific standards for being accepted as such (we will discuss these in detail in Chapter Four). That "experts," be they physicians, teachers, psychologists, counselors, nurses, or anybody else parents trust to help them make decisions in the best interests of their children, continue to perpetuate this fraud is frightening. Equally frightening is that the experts are rewarded for it.

In his book *Raids on the Unspeakable* the Trappist monk, Thomas Merton, wrote an essay called "A Devout Meditation in Memory of Adolf Eichmann" that addressed how Eichmann, who was in charge of transporting Jews and other unwanted minorities to Nazi Germany's concentration camps, could be considered a sane human being despite the obvious horror of what he was participating in. We do not claim that the ADHD fraud is as bad as the Holocaust—the scales are vastly different and cannot be compared. There is, however, a common mechanism that plays a role whenever inhumanity is permitted on a large scale.

> *One of the most disturbing things that came out in the Eichmann trial was that a psychiatrist examined him and pronounced him perfectly sane. I do not doubt it at all, and that is precisely why I find it disturbing.*
>
> *If all the Nazis had been psychotics, as some of their leaders probably were, their appalling cruelty would have been in some sense easier to understand. It is much worse to consider this calm, "well-balanced," unperturbed official conscientiously going about his deskwork, his administrative job which happened to be the supervision of mass murder. He was thoughtful, orderly, unimaginative. He had a profound respect for system, for law and order. He was obedient, loyal, a faithful officer of a great state. He served his government very well.*

Today, our children are subject to educational and health care professionals who advocate the labeling and drugging of normal children. They are conscientious, obedient people who serve the institutions that pay them and provide prestige, security, and opportunities for advancement as well. They are operating with blinders on, to be sure, but they are sane people who would be horrified at the thought of participating in a massive abuse of children. Each individual's part in it is small, with plenty of built-in, rational-sounding justifications for doing what they do. That does not change the result, or excuse it.

It is strange that, while few people advocate for more humane treatment of children in regard to psychiatric abuse, plenty become aroused when animals are similarly abused. For example, a few years ago there was a polar bear named Snowball in the Toronto zoo who looked uncomfortable and unhappy in his cage and was pacing around. After being given Prozac he appeared much happier and sat quietly, no longer pacing. Animal rights activists gathered and protested at the zoo because they didn't like that Snowball had been turned into a docile caged animal. Snowball was taken off Prozac. In America, schools resist children being taken off behavior modifying drugs, no matter how serious the ill effects. If only they treated children with the humanity extended to a zoo animal.

Below is the statement of September 29, 2000, from Patricia Weathers, speaking during a Congressional inquiry into schools pushing ADHD drugs. As frightening as it is, what she and her son were put through is not unusual; what might be unusual is that the school's bullying did not succeed for long. Like Snowball, this boy was drugged because he had trouble adapting to an unnatural and restrictive environment. Why wasn't anybody protesting outside of his school?

STATEMENT OF PATRICIA WEATHERS

My name is Patricia Weathers. I am here to tell you about the ordeal my family has been through and particularly of my son Michael.

When Michael was in kindergarten, we began getting reports that Michael was having behavior problems. Michael was talking out of turn, clowning around in class, and apparently being disruptive. Then when Michael was in the first grade his teacher told me that his learning development was not normal, and that he would not be able to learn unless he was put on medication. Then near the end of first grade the school principal took me into her office and said that unless I agreed to put Michael on psychiatric drugs the school would transfer him to a special education center for children with behavior problems. As a parent I felt extremely pressured by the school's staff at this point. The teacher, school psychologist, principal were all telling me that putting my son on drugs was the right thing to do.

At this point, Michael's first grade teacher filled out an ADHD checklist on Michael and sent it to his pediatrician. Based on this ADHD checklist and a short evaluation by the pediatrician, Michael was given the diagnosis of ADHD and put on the drug Ritalin. According to his teacher Michael was much better, meaning that he was quiet and doing his work.

I didn't notice any difference at first, but eventually I began getting reports that Michael was not socializing with other kids, and that he was withdrawn. This was completely out of character for Michael who was normally very social and outgoing. It got worse. When Michael was in the third grade, my grandmother saw Michael just standing by himself at the far corner of the playground staring at his feet. I also began receiving reports that Michael had started chewing on things, pencils, erasers, and paper, even his clothing. His behavior was getting more and more bizarre.

Instead of recognizing the effects the drugs were having on my son, the school's psychologist claimed Michael now had a social anxiety disorder and needed to see a psychiatrist. She immediately produced the name and the number of the psychiatrist I was to call. The psychiatrist talked to Michael for 15 minutes and, again, with the aid of school reports, diagnosed him with social anxiety disorder. She handed me a prescription for an antidepressant and told me it was a wonder drug for kids.

On October 5, 1999, Michael started taking the antidepressant. Shortly afterwards, he told his teacher he was hearing a male voice in his head telling him to do bad things. I watched as my son began to have wild mood swings and would see him just flip out over the smallest things. One night I tried to get him to just sit down for dinner, and he ran at me in the hallway and attacked me. I could no longer recognize my own son, and I realized it was the drugs that had changed him.

At this point, I did what I knew I had to do. I took him off all drugs. It took him a full month before he stopped hallucinating. The psychiatrist, meanwhile, not recognizing that my son was in withdrawal from a powerful drug, tried to get me to hospitalize him and try different sedatives until I found, "the right one."

The school's psychologist tried to convince me it was "trial and error" in finding the right drug. By now, I was furious and frustrated. I remember I had seen a doctor on TV discussing the drugging of children and how she believed in finding underlying physical causes that could affect a child's behavior. I began doing my own research on these mental disorders, the drugs and their side effects.

In January 2000, I brought my research to the school's psychologist to show her what I believe were the side effects of the medications. The next day I had a meeting with the school staff and the principal. The principal produced my research, then threw it on the desk and said, "I take serious offense over this biased literature." He then told me they had nothing left there to offer my son, and Michael was dismissed from school.

Essentially, this led to a downward chain of events, which culminated in the school calling Child Protective Services on my husband and me, charging us with medical neglect. The charge was for failing to give Michael the necessary medication and failure to follow the psychiatrist's advice of hospitalization. The only reason my son was not removed from my custody that day was that I had obtained an independent psychological evaluation in which the psychologist stated that Michael did not require hospitalization. If it were not for this, he would have been taken from our home.

What concerns me is the intimidation tactics that a school can use to coerce a parent to drug their child. The question is raised, what will happen to the parent without the financial means to combat these tactics? If I didn't have family members who were willing to financially back my son and I in my son's cause, it is entirely possible that my son would have ended up in a psychiatric ward.

Today, Michael is doing fine. He has been off drugs for 9 months and is once again a happy, outgoing boy. He is in a private school, and I also home school him.

***

At the time the school began pressuring Patricia, she was a single parent who they made feel intimidated, scared, and unsure. Trying to do what was best for her son, she found herself ganged up on and badgered. This, sadly, is another unpleasant practice that is not unusual. It is our experience that children from single parent families, from households experiencing any kind of dysfunction, kids in foster care, or any other situation that leaves them more vulnerable than a two-parent household with plenty of time and money to devote to their children, are preyed on as easy targets.

So where did this ADHD diagnosis come from? What could set off a collective madness that continues to grow even as it becomes less sane and more dangerous? An accidental discovery, which we'll tell you about in the next chapter.

Chapter Three

EVOLUTION OF AN EPIDEMIC:
A Drug in Search of a Disease

I say again that the thing that troubles me is that we are about to embark on a program placing millions of children on drugs we know so little about.

> —Congressman Cornelius Gallagher (NJ), presiding over the House of Representatives Special Studies Subcommittee on Government Operations, at a hearing on Federal involvement in the use of behavior modification drugs on grammar school children, September 29, 1970 [1]

I would first like to point out that every drug, however innocuous, has some degree of toxicity. A drug, therefore, is a type of poison and its poisonous qualities must be carefully weighed against its therapeutic usefulness. A problem now being considered in most of the capitals of the free world is whether the benefits derived from amphetamines outweigh their toxicity. It is the consensus of the world scientific literature that the amphetamines are of little benefit to mankind. They are, however, quite toxic.

> —Dr. John Griffith, Professor of Psychiatry, Vanderbilt University, testifying at the same hearing

The discovery that amphetamines could be used to alter the behavior of children was made by accident in 1937. Charles Bradley was a physician at the Emma Pendleton Bradley Home in Rhode Island, a residential treatment center for children diagnosed with behavioral and neurological disorders. He observed the "calming" effect of stimulants on children when he gave Benzedrine (trademark for amphetamine) to a group of 30 children in order to treat headaches that resulted from spinal taps they were given. The Benzedrine did not do anything for the headaches, but it did make the children less active and more compliant, in a fashion he called "spectacular."

In a chilling preview of the epidemic to come, he reported, "to see a single dose of Benzedrine produce a greater improvement in school performance than the combined efforts of a capable staff working in a most favorable setting, would have been all but demoralizing to the teachers had not the improvement been so gratifying from a practical viewpoint." In the years that followed this anecdotal observation that stimulants have this effect was further reinforced and sparked the manufacture of both more drugs and the rationales necessary to justify giving them to troublesome children everywhere.

Nobody is going to come out and say that children should be forced to take speed and drugged into submission for the real reasons—it makes dealing with unruly children easier and a hugely profitable market exists for anything that can accomplish that feat. A diagnosible abnormality needed to be invented in order to provide the appearance of legitimate "treatment" being rendered in their best interests.

When Bradley further stated that, "It appears paradoxical that a drug known to be a stimulant should produce subdued behavior," he gave seed to the root of a misconception that continues to persist today, namely, that stimulants given to children labeled as ADHD affects them differently than normal people. The hope was that this would be so because a different reaction to the drugs could be used to help support the notion that there really was something wrong with the brains of ADHD labeled children that did not occur in the heads of normal kids. As further study revealed, however, these drugs have the same impact on just about anybody who gets them. The idea that something paradoxical was going on came from the fact that the "low" doses of amphetamines given to children increased their ability to focus on repetitive tasks and be compliant, just as happens to adults. It is at higher dosage levels that the effects more commonly associated with amphetamines (speed) occur.

In 1950 Dr. Bradley did another study with children, using Benzedrine (amphetamine) and Dexedrine (dextro-amphetamine). Of the 275 children given these, he reported between 60% and 70% to be much improved while on the drugs. Much improved meaning, as it does today, that their behavior became more appealing according to adult standards while under the influence of addictive drugs.

A DRUG IN SEARCH OF A DISEASE

The best known of the stimulants given to children, methylphenidate (Ritalin), was synthesized by Ciba (a pharmaceutical company that later morphed into Novartis) in 1944, with its pharmacology described in 1954. In his excellent book, *The Creation of Psychopharmacology*, David Healy, M.D., [2] tells us, "Later Leon Eisenberg used Ritalin in the first randomized controlled trial involving children, to test its effects on hyperactive states. It was effective and its effectiveness led to the acceptance of the concept of minimal brain dysfunction, which in 1980 in DSM-III [3] became attention deficit disorder (ADD). Since then a growing, almost epidemic, use of Ritalin to treat this condition has become headline news."

Note the extremely important point made above by Healy; it was the drug's effectiveness that lead to the acceptance of minimal brain dysfunction, the parent to ADD and ADHD. The fact that Ritalin worked in the same way on a particular group of children as it would on anybody was used to promote a diagnosis targeted at specific groups of (normal) children it claimed, as proponents of ADHD do today, had malfunctioning brains, as evidenced by their response to drug treatment. Is this just bad reasoning? Or was a deliberately deceitful strategy hatched to create patients and drug consumers where none should have existed?

The earliest precursor of ADHD came in the early 1900s when children who were unusually active, impulsive, or rebellious, might be diagnosed as having minimal brain damage, a term coined by Dr. George Still. The idea was that since brain damage can cause changes in behavior these children may have suffered some kind of assault on their brains. Indeed, a variety of conditions that damage the brain are associated with difficulties in attention and heightened activity levels, such as fetal alcohol syndrome or lead poisoning, but there is no meaningful correlation between known brain injuries or diseases in children and the inability to pay attention, sit still, or regulate one's impulses.

The minimal brain dysfunction label that came after Eisenberg's study of Ritalin removed the assumption of an injury to the brain and replaced it with the notion that something in the heads of these children was amiss, their brains somehow misfiring due to an abnormality they were born with, though nobody ever figured out what, or exactly where in the brain, it was. It was pure speculation with never a shred of scientific evidence to back it up. Hyperkinetic reaction was another label used in the 50s and 60s, though it never specified what was being reacted to and was simply a label for an active child in whom nothing verifiably wrong had been found.

In 1979 the Food and Drug Administration ordered that minimal brain dysfunction be eliminated as a diagnostic term. They banished it because MBD was unscientific (had no grounding in facts). With symptoms of it no different than normal childhood behaviors, the diagnosis was rightly banished. Unfortunately, one bad idea was replaced by a worse idea, the creation of ADD, still completely unscientific but said to be an improvement because its diagnostic criteria were expanded and seemingly more specific. What this really did, however, was make it possible to include even more typical childhood behaviors under the diagnostic umbrella so that millions of normal children could be diagnosed and billions of dollars could be made off needlessly drugging them.

During the days of minimal brain dysfunction and hyperkinetic reaction the fields of psychology and psychiatry generally regarded children's problems as stemming from their environments, primarily as the result of faulty parenting. No matter what emotional or behavioral problems beset a person, so the reasoning went, the cause could be found in something that had gone wrong, or was going wrong, in childhood. Individuals were regarded as being in possession of naturally healthy brains, with rare exceptions of those with conspicuous brain damage, and only experienced psychological difficulties as the result of unhealthy experiences.

In this kind of climate, viewing the behavioral problems of a child as being the result of defects within his own brain was a rare thing, which is why relatively few children were diagnosed with minimal brain dysfunction, or given behavior-modifying drugs. Things began to change late in the 60s, with a major shift obvious by the beginning of the 80s. Increasingly, psychiatry became a discipline where behavioral problems were seen as having biological rather than environmental roots, even though no proofs were ever produced for this shift in thinking. Now chemical imbalances and other forms of neurological abnormalities became the fashionable explanations. The contradiction right from the beginning was that, even though psychiatry increasingly claimed a biological basis for behavioral disorders, the discipline never produced any biological evidence to support its contentions. On one hand, psychiatry claims to be scientific, but on the other it has never produced evidence that passes scientific muster. What psychiatry has is a set of unsupported assumptions we are told to accept on faith, until the always-promised proof is discovered. In effect we are told to wait, like Charlie Brown sitting through the night in hopes of the Great Pumpkin's arrival.

Along with a different outlook on behavioral causes, in the past there was more understanding and tolerance for the normal range of childhood behaviors. Children vary greatly in interests, abilities, talents, and behavioral styles and this was commonly known and understood, as it is today when we choose to be reasonable about it. In the years since, with all the talk of diversity and the acceptance of differences among individuals, the tolerance for differences in how children act has plummeted. It used to be that the child who did poorly academically was understood to be somebody who would excel in other areas, where things like physical talent, creativity, personal skills, and the ability to switch gears quickly were called for, not the ability to sit still and obey directives.

In 1961 Ritalin was approved by the Food and Drug Administration for use in children and remained, by today's standards, a drug not often employed, with the number of children taking it in 1970 being approximately 150,000. How did it go from that relatively low number to the over 6 million children today being given Ritalin and a variety of amphetamines? Lots of factors are involved, but the most obvious turning point came when schools began devoting themselves to identifying candidates for chemical restraint. And, as educators got better at it, psychiatry joined in by broadening the diagnostic criteria to the point where almost any child could be targeted for behavior modifying drugs. Along with them, pharmaceutical companies were quick to catch on to the huge market for stimulant drugs and went to great lengths to market the "disease" and their treatments for it. In speaking of pharmaceutical companies, Dr. Healy points out that they have gone from barely existing prior to World War II to become "...giant corporations and the darlings of Wall Street...a medico-pharmaceutical complex that appears to have gradually shifted from discovering treatments for major diseases to medicalizing aspects of the human condition. We live in a Brave New World which is shaped not just by new drugs created in company laboratories, but by an almost Orwellian capacity to control the flow of information."

Since 1970, parents have been flooded by misinformation from their schools, psychiatry, ADHD support groups, and the pharmaceutical companies, all telling them that even small deviations from narrow standards of behavior are evidence of a disease within the child, when none are—not a single one. Parents are also told these drugs are mild, safe, and effective. Of the two, the "disease" lie is absolute, in and of itself, abrogating the patient's right to informed consent.

It is interesting to note that as the definitions of, and criteria for MBD, ADD, and ADHD, were changed over the years, they became broader instead of more specific. How much of this was driven by the expanding knowledge of the impact of stimulants on children's behavior? Need one be paranoid to suspect that the diagnosis was broadened to accommodate a treatment that would "work" across the board?

Normally, as a condition is studied and more is learned about it, the diagnostic signs (signs=objective abnormalities) are narrowed down to a specific set of objective criteria that can be reliably applied. With ADHD the opposite happened, with more and more behaviors thrown into this free-for-all stew so that now it has become possible to pretty much drug any child who is not behaving or performing precisely as those with power over him want.

In their excellent book, [4] *Coping with Children's Temperament*, William Carey, M.D., and Sean McDevitt, Ph.D., go into some of the problems with the ADHD label, saying "...our view is that the term ADHD is commonly used in the United States today to refer to an oversimplified grouping of a complex and variable set of normal but incompatible temperament variations, disabilities in cognition, problems in school function and behavior, and sometimes neurological immaturities. We believe that many different conditions are being called by this one name." If there is ever to be a legitimate label to denote a problem with attention, activity, or impulsivity, it will have to be much more specific and refer to a physical abnormality that can be identified objectively. This, after all, is the definition of disease.

Carey and McDevitt talk about "when" ADHD is identified. But, precisely because the diagnostic criteria for ADHD (which we will examine in specific detail in Chapter 5), are comprised of normal childhood behaviors, we see no reason for this optimism. If any true disease were to be discovered and verified that interferes with a child's ability to pay attention, control her activity levels, or reign in her impulsivity, it will have a scientific basis and objective means of identification. However, the American Psychiatric Association's, DSM (Diagnostic and Statistical Manual) process of cobbling together subjective symptoms, voting on them, and calling them "diseases," bears no resemblance to the discovery of unique, new abnormalities (abnormality = disease) by observant physicians, and will never validate ADHD or any other psychiatric "disorder" as an actual disease. [5] [6]

In the meantime, if a nonscientific diagnosis for ADHD is going to continue on, it should at least be modified to reflect the real problem, which lies solely in adults. As a guide to this reality upgrade, we present the tongue-in-cheek quote below, from the pediatrician Daniel Zeidner in a letter published in the journal *Pediatrics* in 1995:

> *It has become increasingly apparent to me, and perhaps to other pediatricians, that a new syndrome exists among adults who teach our school-aged children: Teacher Deficit Disorder, or TDD. I have observed that this diagnosis should be made on the teacher when the following classic signs and symptoms exist among one or more of his/her students: students who fidget in class constantly moving their arms or legs, who do not pay attention, who frequently daydream, who do not complete their homework or classwork, and who frequently get out of their seats. When students exhibit these manifestations, the teacher should be diagnosed with TDD, and, of course, should be medicated immediately with amphetamine or other drugs that would speed him/her up, thus making him/her...more dynamic and interesting to his/her students.*

PREVIEW OF THE PLAGUE

For anybody wishing a detailed blueprint of how American schools came to be the most successful drug pushers in the land, the Gallagher Report is essential reading. The bulk of it records a hearing conducted by a subcommittee of the House of Representatives on September 29, 1970, [7] into what its chairman, Representative Cornelius Gallagher, described in his opening statement as "...our hearing into Federal responsibility in promoting the use of amphetamines to modify the behavior of grammar school children."

The hearings were the result of concerns over almost $3 million in federal funds spent by the National Institute of Mental Health on research grants for the study of learning disabilities, with every funded study including the use of drugs on children who were identified as being afflicted with minimal brain dysfunction. He articulated his concerns very well, describing, "The problem of labeling so many hundreds of thousands of our children where there has in fact been no medical diagnosis of that child, other than to make the child's attention span a little broader than it has been. If this is the trend, we may be supporting it by federal grants. It would seem to me we are about to do a great disservice to a great number of children." He also expressed concern about the developing roles of schools in spreading what has now become a worldwide epidemic: "the other trouble is that in the educational societies themselves they are becoming aware of the uses of behavior modification programs."

Another premonition of things to come came from a chemist testifying at the hearings. One of his concerns was the lack of scientific objectivity found in studies of the stimulants used in the treatment of children. Like Dr. David Healy years later, who we quoted earlier in the chapter and will again in forthcoming pages, he was troubled by the sources of information that were relied upon by physicians, parents, and educators (who never had any business in the process to begin with) when deciding whether or not to administer stimulants to children. "A critical search through the literature will very likely reveal that 90 percent or more of the research, evaluation, and presentation of these drugs was conducted by the drug companies, or through investigations underwritten by the companies." This trend has continued, indeed, become worse in the years since, as the flow of information has become increasingly under the control of those who stand to gain the greatest financial rewards. Is this who we want educating our doctors? Our teachers? Deciding what drugs our children are required to take?

Today, at a time when tens of millions of children worldwide have been diagnosed with ADHD and are being forced to take an array of powerful drugs, it is fascinating to look back see such concern for 150,000 children being similarly abused. What Representative Gallagher correctly feared was that, as bad as it was to target that number of children, the future was only going to get worse. If only he had been wrong.

Not only did Gallagher have a sense of the dangers of the drugs being administered, he astutely saw the threat such diagnostic and doping practices represented to childhood itself. "From the time of puberty onward, each and every child is told that 'speed kills' and that amphetamines are to be avoided. Yet, this same child has learned that Ritalin, for example, is the only thing which makes him a functioning member of the school environment and both his family and his doctor have urged the pills on him." Soon after the above statement, Gallagher went on to add:

> I am well aware of the occasional frustrations which come from the fact that children do not simply sit quietly and perform assigned tasks. Based on my personal experience, I believe that children learn with all their senses, not just with their eyes and ears. For childhood is an exploratory time and the great energy of children propels them into situations which may look frivolous or counterproductive to more restrained adults, but which are the sum and substance of the child's learning experience. I do not think I am overstating the case when I say

*that the learning environment for the young child is the total
environment and every experience is a learning experience.
Obviously, this unstructured passion for all the events in a
child's world is regarded as unruly and disruptive, particularly in overcrowded classrooms. I fear that there is a very
great temptation to diagnose the bored but bright child as
hyperactive, prescribe drugs, and thus deny him full learning
during his most creative years.*

In retrospect, it appears that the studies being conducted may
well have been designed with the aim of producing "evidence" of
the effectiveness of drugs (primarily Ritalin at the time) in the
treatment of minimal brain dysfunction. As we mention time and
time again in this book, Ritalin and other stimulants do alter behavior in ways schools find favorable, so manufacturing data to
support their effectiveness would not be a difficult thing.

This becomes very apparent when a pro-drugging child psychiatrist who testified, Dr. John Peters, had this to say about how
kids acted before the drugs were administered, "The experiences
of these children prior to medication are distressing—inability to
attend to what the teacher is saying, or to concentrate on the page
in front of them; inability to resist talking out in class or answering
constantly whether called upon or not; inability to tolerate waiting their turn in the classroom or on the playground; a feeling of
restlessness and out-of-control driven-ness." Any drug that quiets
these behaviors and enhances the ability to focus can be regarded
as a good thing. What Dr. Peters does here is precisely what continues to this day, to make a disease out of childhood. Nowhere
does he mention that maybe this is how kids have always acted,
that maybe the classroom and teacher are dull, that just maybe
the children would respond better if the adults around them did a
better job. To him and the legions of his ilk, a troublesome child
is a diseased child. Another committee member brought up an
excellent point in response by saying, "If you read all the good
results of giving these children drugs you wonder, maybe if you
gave every child a little bit of it, they might all be better off. They
might all become more docile or more cooperative or something

of this nature. This would almost seem to follow logically from what you are driving at here." Indeed it does.

Back in 1970 we see that the schools were already beginning to resort to powerful drugs to control children rather than developing better methods of running classrooms. Some have said the turn to drugs came as a result of the banishing of physical punishments in schools, but are schools really so limited that they can't control children without weapons, be they a hand, paddle, or drug? [8]

Susan B. Anthony, leader of the women's suffrage movement and a teacher herself, put it well by saying, "I taught little children six hours a day and got $1 a week and my board. Oh, my yes! I whipped lots of them. As I got older I abolished whipping. If I could not manage a child, I thought it my ignorance or my lack of ability as a teacher." If only educators in the 70s had developed this attitude instead of an increasing fondness for drugs as tools of classroom management.

Gallagher addressed this shift in the approach of schools by stating the following:

> *Federal funds have been used to support various experimental programs and studies concerning the use of drugs to treat learning disabilities in children. Assisted by this infusion of tax dollars, it has become apparent that biochemical mediation and alteration of the learning environment is considered part of a 'new wave' approach to education in the United States by many persons both in and out of government.*

Representative Gallagher also made it clear that this new wave was not the best approach and seriously doubted the appropriateness of using federal dollars to fuel its spread, "...we have seen a dependence on quick and inexpensive solutions ordered by the new technology without adequate attention being paid to the slower and perhaps more costly methods which would preserve the sanctity of human values and the precious resources of the human spirit."

* * *

Despite the relatively small number of children being medicated for MBD in 1970, a psychiatrist testifying at the Gallagher hearing estimated that 3 - 10% of children under 12 years of age had MBD. A CIBA (the manufacturer of Ritalin then) catalog quoted from at the hearing estimated that 5% or more of children had it. Even more disturbing, the same catalog said that candidates for referral to physicians for evaluation should be identified by teachers, counselors, nurses, and school psychologists. Here we have a *drug manufacturer* proposing that school personnel generate business for them! In the years since, schools have done just that in their eagerness for the payoff they get in return—easier-to-manage children.

Representative Gallagher was also prophetic in his concern that increasing numbers of children would be forced to take drugs so similar to those schools tell them to avoid, namely, speed and cocaine. Today millions of dollars are spent on DARE, the drug prevention program run in schools across the country. Though study after study has shown DARE to be completely ineffective (kids who go through the program are no less likely to abuse drugs than those who do not), schools insist on maintaining the program. At the same time they persist in their futile efforts at drug abuse prevention, they continue to push drugs on ever more children for an ever-increasing list of invented psychiatric disorders. When Gallagher said, "The thing that really troubles me in this is a certain glibness about the experimentation on young children in this country, used as guinea pigs," he articulated a concern that has only become more serious in the years since 1970.

Representative Gallagher was not the only prophetic speaker at the hearings. An associate of John Holt, an educational consultant and lecturer at Harvard, read a statement he'd prepared for the committee. Mr. Holt was raising the point that something other than brain damage might be causing children to act in undesirable ways at school. Note how true the words ring today. Note also how they have been largely ignored by our schools and those physicians who prescribe stimulants for children so glibly.

> *Might not one of the causes be the fact that we take lively, curious, energetic children, eager to make contact with the world and to learn about it, stick them in barren classrooms with teachers who on the whole neither like nor respect nor understand nor trust them, restrict their freedom of speech and movement to a degree that would be judge excessive and inhuman even in a maximum security prison, and that their teachers themselves could not and would not tolerate? Then, when the children resist this brutalizing and stupefying treatment and retreat from it in anger, bewilderment, and terror, we say that they are sick with 'complex and little-understood' disorders, and proceed to dose them with powerful drugs that are indeed complex and of whose long-run effects we know little or nothing, so that they may be more ready to do the asinine things the schools ask them to do.*

The only thing that has changed from what was said above in 1970 is that schools have become far more aggressive in initiating the process of getting troublesome children chemically restrained, with physicians, parents, and everybody else going right along. Whoever wrote that CIBA catalog exhorting school personnel to drum up business for Ritalin could never have dreamed how effective these legions of drug pushers would become, nor the billions of dollars in revenues to come.

Mr. Holt's statement goes on to demonstrate an understanding of children we can only wish were present in classrooms, counseling offices, and examining rooms:

> *Children have a great deal of energy; they like to move about; they live and learn with their bodies and muscles, not just their eyes and ears; when adults try to compel them to remain still and silent for long periods of time they resent and resist it; most of them can be cowed and silenced by various bribes and*

*threats; 5 to 15 percent cannot. These we diagnose as suffering
from a 'learning malady called hyperkinesis.'*

Another of the wonderful things highlighted here is that not
every child is a candidate for chemical constraining, just that portion of children who are resistant (though the number judged to
be in this group has steadily grown). Holt knew, back in 1970, that
hyperkinesis and minimal brain dysfunction, the forerunners of
ADD and ADHD, were not diseases at all, just collections of irritating behaviors that were grouped together to form a diagnosis
that could be used to justify medicating these traits away.

*We consider it a disease because it makes it difficult to run our
schools as we do, like maximum security prisons, for the comfort and convenience of the teachers and administrators who
work in them. The energy of children is 'bad' because it is a
nuisance to the exhausted and overburdened adults who do not
want to or know how to and are not able to keep up with it.*
  *Given the fact that some children are more energetic and ac-
tive than others, might it not be easier, more healthy, and more
humane to deal with this fact by giving them more time and
scope to make use of and work off their energy?*

Below is a story from a parent who testified at the Gallagher
hearing, having had an experience at the hands of her children's
school system way back in the 60s that will sound very familiar
to parents of today. It reveals the relentless pressure parents are
subject to when their child has been identified as a candidate for
chemical restraint. In addressing the practice during the hearing,
Gallagher said, "...that brings the whole referral system under
question and it causes one to wonder how a teacher or an administrator can continually call and harass a parent..." Part of
this harassment typically involves direct referral to a drug or a
strong push when drugs are not specifically mentioned, a practice
Gallagher had this to say about: "Whether they identify the drug
by its name, such as Ritalin, or whether they say this child needs
to be placed on a tranquilizer before I will teach him again, this

amounts to coercion, when you consider the relationship of the average parent to such an authoritative person as a teacher."

Although schools did not really hit their stride with pushing the ADHD diagnosis and drugs until the late 80s, testimony at the Gallagher Hearings reveals that it began back in the sixties. Below is a summary of the testimony of one mother, providing us a chilling look at what so many more families were to experience at the hands of their schools.

BACK TO THE FUTURE

Mrs. Youngs and her husband and two children lived in Little Rock, Arkansas from 1963 until 1966. During that time both children were singled out by the school as candidates for the diagnosis of minimal brain dysfunction and drug treatment. Representative Cornelius Gallagher (NJ), when introducing Mrs. Youngs to the committee said, "The testimony is indicative of many other experiences of parents in the rest of the country."

The whole mess started in the fall of 1963, when Mrs. Youngs and her husband went to their new school and enrolled their third-grade daughter and first-grade son. During a meeting with the school principal, she studied the children's report cards (brought by the parents) for a few minutes, and then said to them, "Your daughter, Mr. and Mrs. Youngs, has minimal brain damage." She went on to share that her own daughter had minimal brain dysfunction, too, and was taking drugs to stimulate her learning. The Youngs studied the literature the principal gave them on minimal brain dysfunction and found more material in the library. They concluded that, "It was absolutely insane to give children with average and above average intelligence amphetamines and other drugs to stimulate their learning capacity."

Their daughter had difficulty reading at her grade level, which inspired the principal to continue urging that the girl be tested and medicated, saying that she was underactive and a daydreamer. "During the school year of 1963-64, I was called constantly and went down for conference after conference about my daughter, always about the same thing—minimal brain dysfunction—and always with the same result. We would not cooperate with their program." Their children got Bs and Cs that year and the next year. Still, "During the school year of 1964-65 I was called down to the school at least once a week about my daughter and son. I was told my son was overactive and my daughter underactive."

The 1965-1966 school year started off well, with the Youngs feeling relieved because they didn't hear anything from the school during the first month, but the badgering started up again in October. Within the same week Mrs. Youngs was asked to come in for conferences with her son's teacher and her daughter's teacher. "My daughter's teacher was saying the same thing I had heard for 2 years—have your daughter tested for minimal brain dysfunction. At the conference with my son's teacher I heard these words for the first time: 'Mrs. Youngs, I think your son has minimal brain dysfunction and we would like to test him.' When Mrs. Youngs went down the hall to complain to the principal, she was told the school was considering testing both children with or without consent.

The parents received notes almost daily for the next few months. "We were told our children had completely quit trying and were failing every subject."

Their son was not allowed to have recess with other children. One day he came home crying hysterically. "He had been put in a cardboard box for 2 weeks."

The box was gone when Mrs. Youngs went to the school to complain, though she was told that some parents were going to build wooden partitions. The idea behind both the box and the partitions was to eliminate distractions for children judged not to be attentive enough, though it is hard to imagine any teacher putting a boy in a box without realizing that the psychological damage of being thrust into a box in a room full of one's peers would surely outweigh any benefits.

Early in 1966 Mrs. Youngs took her son to their family physician for a routine visit. During the exam their doctor asked how he was doing in school. The boy replied, "I get Cs and Ds." Then the doctor asked her son "how he would like it if he could get As and Bs. My son said he would like that." The doctor wrote out a prescription for stimulant drugs and told the child they would help him do better. Mrs. Youngs refused the prescription and found a new physician.

Near the end of the school year the principal called Mrs. Youngs in for yet another meeting, where she informed her that both children were failing and, since the parents weren't doing anything about it, the school was considering legal action to force the issue of "diagnosis." [9] Before things came to that the Youngs family moved to Indiana. Testifying at the 1970 hearings with her children, now 15 and 13, Mrs. Youngs testified that her daughter was now an A and B student and her son a B and C student.

FROM ATTACKS ON INDIVIDUAL CHILDREN TO AN ATTACK ON CHILDHOOD ITSELF

Despite minimal brain damage being removed as a diagnosis by the FDA in 1979 because it was unscientific, it did not take long before it was replaced by a construct even less scientific. Attention Deficit Disorder made its debut in 1980, appearing in the third edition of the *Diagnostic and Statistical Manual*, a diagnostic guide published by the American Psychiatric Association and updated every few years.

With ADD the emphasis switched from activity levels, as were dominant with hyperkinetic disorder and minimal brain damage, and focused on problems of inattentiveness. Attention Deficit Disorder could be diagnosed with or without hyperactivity. The basic ADD diagnosis could be made if a child exhibited several behaviors from two groups of possible choices. The first group was for inattentiveness; the second for impulsivity. Both

menus contained a lot of overlap, as the ADHD diagnosis continues to today, so a child did not have to display wide-ranging
evidence of an impairment in order to be diagnosed. Just being
distractible, not seeming to listen, or failing to finish tasks was
enough to qualify for the inattentiveness group, while interrupting, not taking turns, talking at the wrong time, and a few more
similar sins, made up the selections from the impulsivity group. In
order to achieve a diagnosis of ADD with hyperactivity, several
items from a third group had to be present, things like climbing,
running, and appearing to be "driven by a motor."

Notice that right from the beginning of its tenure in the
DSM, ADD was heavily weighted toward behaviors that put children in conflict with school personnel. The groups of behaviors
were considered to be symptoms. As you recall from our earlier
discussion of disease, symptoms are subjective and are not, by
themselves, enough to make a diagnosis, they must be accompanied by signs—abnormalities—that can be objectively verified
(through physical examination, blood tests, scans, x-rays, etc.)
as abnormalities before a disease can be diagnosed. With ADD,
all that was required for a diagnosis was the presence of enough
symptoms whose severity, or even existence, is completely subjective. This is also why it became so easy for teachers, counselors,
psychologists and the like to make claims that ADD existed in a
child. Anybody can observe a symptom, especially if the symptoms are identical to normal behaviors. For ADD, childhood
itself became the pathology.

In 1987 the revised 3rd edition of the DSM (DSM-III-R) [10]
appeared and it featured a new version of ADD. The emphasis on
high activity levels had returned and the name was broadened to
accommodate the change, now becoming attention deficit/hyper-
activity disorder. Instead of three groups to choose from, there
was now one list of 14 symptoms, of which any eight could be
observed in order to make the diagnosis. It was claimed that the
new ADHD criteria were the result of extensive field trials, as
had been said about ADD seven years earlier. The truth is that

no legitimate scientific research ever underlay ADD or ADHD, a fact that continues to this day. ADD was voted into existence by a committee of psychiatrists and psychologists, as was ADHD in 1987 and the last version in the 1994 DSM-IV. [11] In effect, all manifestations of the disorder (by which they meant disease) simply came into existence because their respective committees said so. They voted to make a disease out of childhood.

Here are the 14 symptoms that appeared in 1987 *Diagnostic and Statistical Manual*:

1. often fidgets or squirms (feelings of rest lessness in adolescents of adults).

2. difficulty remaining seated.

3. easily distracted by extraneous stimuli.

4. difficulty awaiting turn.

5. often blurts out answers before questions have been completed.

6. difficulty following through on instructions or finishing chores (not due to oppositional behavior or difficulty comprehending).

7. difficulty sustaining attention.

8. often shifts from one uncompleted activity to another.

9. difficulty playing quietly.

10. often talks excessively.

11. often interrupts or intrudes.

12. often does not seem to listen.

13. often loses things necessary for tasks or activities.

14. often does dangerous things without considering consequences (not for thrill seeking).

After reading through the list one can only be left with the conclusion that the field trials conducted to develop ADHD consisted of going out and observing normal children and making a list of things that irritate adults who do not possess the patience, compassion, or interest to tolerate them. As all of us who are parents know that children can be irritating, but that does not mean there is any reason to medicalize the traits that bug us.

In 1994 4th edition of the DSM (DSM-IV) the version of ADHD currently in use was published. This one reverted to something closer to the 1980 version with a renewed emphasis on problems of attention. It will not be reviewed here because the DSM IV criteria for ADHD are looked at closely in Chapter 5. Each generation of ADD/ADHD mandated that it be a chronic pattern of behavior in existence before age seven (not a hard condition to meet, as children remain children before and after the age of seven) and had to manifest itself to a greater degree than seen in most people of the same mental age. Never is it made clear when the "greater degree" is achieved or how to determine "mental age," evidence of the same lack of clarity or credibility that runs rampant throughout ADHD and makes it possible to brand any child, except maybe those who have already been trained to act like adults, God help them, with the label.

Despite no evidence of ADHD being a neurobiological syndrome, brain abnormality, chemical imbalance, or disease of any kind, the numbers of children diagnosed with it has rocketed from 150,000 in 1970, to 500,000 in 1980, to over 6 million today. From 1990 to 1997 annual production of Ritalin increased by 700%, and this was at a time when competing drugs were being introduced. Most horrifying of all is the 500,000 or so children between the ages of 2–5 now being treated with powerful drugs for ADHD. Nobody has any idea of the effects these drugs will have on children so young. Dr. Joseph Coyle, Chairman of Psychiatry at Harvard Medical School, commented in the February 23, 2000 New York Times that, "These interventions are occurring at a critical time in brain development, and we don't know what the consequences are." [12] That we are willing to tolerate this is unfathomable.

Though psychiatry has certainly been a guilty party in the promotion of medicating ever more and ever younger children, other physicians who work with them, like pediatricians, neurologists, and family practitioners, take part also. A *U.S. News & World Report* article spoke of doctors who complain that they are "pressured by managed-care companies and insurers to avoid referring their patients to mental health specialists and to reduce the time they spend with families." Indeed, reduce the time spent with a child they have. According to Harold Koplewicz in a February 23, 2000 article at Salon.com, "The average pediatrician sees a child for seven and a half minutes. A good diagnosis of a behavioral problem requires at least one and a half hours." Being pressured unduly is not a nice experience, but neither is it a nice experience for a child to be unduly drugged as a result.

The real surge in ADHD diagnosing came after 1980, when the DSM could be used to give it the appearance of medical validity and an excuse for prescribing drugs under cover of the false disease pretense. Decades of research have failed to provide any support for the validity of ADHD, yet, the fact that is a contrived illusion of a disease has not slowed down its spread a bit.

The psychiatric illusions of disease have spread, not just in the amount ascribed to a particular disorder, but in the range of disorders (diseases) children are being diagnosed with. Today, in addition to ADHD, we have upwards of 2 million children diagnosed and actively drugged for things like anxiety disorders and bi-polar disorder and, just like with ADHD, there is no proof they exist as diseases, syndromes, have pathologies, an etiology, reside in the brain, or anything else. They are nothing but predatory inventions.

DRUGS R US: A PILL FOR EVERY CHILD

A 2002 survey done by the Yale Child Study Center and published in the *Journal of the American Academy of Child and Adolescent Psychiatry*, found that 9 of 10 children who visit a child psychiatrist will come away with a prescription. As if this is not predatory enough, most of those prescriptions, when they are made for disorders other than ADHD, are for drugs that have never been tested in children or approved for use in children by the Food and Drug Administration. Whether or not the drugs are safe, dangerous, beneficial, or prone to make things worse is simply not known. The practice is called off-label prescribing. Doctors can prescribe a drug for children after it has been approved for use in adults, the assumption being that they will administer it responsibly. As proven by the exponentially swelling ranks of normal children being forced to ingest drugs for unproven disorders, that assumption is no longer warranted.

One of the most incredible things about the ADHD epidemic is that over the years of its evolution all proffered "proofs" have been found false. Not a single benefit of diagnosis or drugging has been found. The numbers of children harmed, both physically and psychologically, continues to mount and, yet, it only gets worse here in the United States and is spreading around the world.

Representative Gallagher provided us a prophetic warning of things to come, and it was ignored. Just as he feared, ever more children who acted like kids in school were labeled and chemically constrained. What nobody could have foreseen was the extent to which the attack on childhood would broaden. Now children who are sad, angry, worried, or acting out in any way can have a variety of labels, in all kinds of combinations, affixed to them. Their behaviors are indeed symptoms of disturbing things, but these things are not diseases brewing in their brains, they are adult dysfunctions in adult-controlled environments that are then visited on children. If anybody is mired in the throes of diseased brains, it is the grown-ups who invent disease after disease in order to profit from the attack on childhood.

Chapter Four

DOLLARS FOR DISEASES

… it appears that you define disease as a maladaptive cluster of characteristics. In the history of science and medicine, this would not be a valid definition of disease.

- Richard Degrandpre, Ph.D., commenting on the Report of the Panel of the November 16-18, 1998, ADHD Consensus Conference

Modern psychiatry has forgotten the Hippocratic principle: Above all, do no harm.

- Loren Mosher, M.D.

When it comes to children and drugs, it is distressing to witness how the efforts made, both in promoting some drugs and discouraging the use of others, serve a variety of interests – with those of children employed mostly as an excuse for agendas that do them no good. For an example, let's take a look at the D.A.R.E. (Drug Abuse Resistance Education) program.

Whenever I (co-author Craig Hovey) go to the elementary school that all three of my children have attended I am struck by the signs out front by the bus loop proclaiming the school a "drug free zone." At mandated times during the year teachers, administrators, and students sport red ribbons on their shirts that are supposed to symbolize a unified front against drug use. In fifth grade every student is shuttled through a D.A.R.E. course, a nationwide program costing billions of dollars that is supposed to educate children to the dangers of illegal drugs and keep them from using any. At the same time though, this elementary school and the suburban district it functions within do their part to en-sure that thousands of children are forced to *take* drugs, which, often times, are barely distinguishable from those D.A.R.E. tells them never to touch. Maybe they are able to keep this suburban bus loop free of drug pushers, but inside the building they violate the bodies of student after student by treating them as zones to be made drug friendly. What is going on here?

The D.A.R.E. program has been shown to be ineffective in study after study. It does no better a job of keeping kids off drugs than if they took no course at all. But D.A.R.E. continues on, eating dollars while producing no real benefits for our children. Schools like it because it gives them the appearance of doing something worthwhile. In short, D.A.R.E. is a feel-good program for deluded adults that wastes the time of children who would profit much more if the resources were devoted to real education.

While D.A.R.E. instructors tell children of the dangers of cocaine and amphetamines, teachers, school psychologists, and administrators continue to see to it that students are forced to take drugs that are either very similar or identical to them. Rit-alin, as mentioned earlier, is quite similar to cocaine, and drugs like Adderall are amphetamine mixtures. In the same classroom a drug can be defined as a horrible substance that should never pass a child's lips at one moment then, when a child has been tar-geted and an unknowing parent set up for an ambush, presented as a wonderful medicine that will save a child from a life of doom, gloom, and failure.

A perplexing paradox? No. The explanation is simple: schools, pharmaceutical companies, medical professionals, and insurance companies like the drugs they profit from and cast them in a positive light accordingly. The pushers who lie beyond the bus loop barricades provide them no profits, even when their wares are very similar. Professional conduct, knowledge, integrity, and ethics are abandoned with nary a look back when the carrots of increased revenues, decreased expenses, a broader patient base, or easier-to-manage children are within biting range, things that yield more profits through increased cash flows seen on financial statements or an increased flow of compliant students in the hallways. At least the pushers of illegal drugs make no pretense about acting for the good of children. At least the pushers of illegal drugs don't claim to treat "diseases." At least the pushers of illegal drugs, don't target infants, toddlers, and preschoolers. [1]

The real disease behind the diagnosis and drugging of children is not being treated at all. In fact, it has been running wild and gaining in power and audacity, encouraged by its own success. And what disease is this? Not a physical disease at all, but more deadly than any of them, a disease that predates the creation of ADHD by many thousands of years, a disease of the human soul and one that no medication stands a chance against. Greed.

For us, maybe the most heartbreaking case of a child and family bearing all the costs while professionals and corporations profited came in the story of Shaina Dunkle. In September of 2002 I visited her parents, Vicky and Steve, in their home in Smethport, Pennsylvania. They showed me Shaina's room, which was preserved exactly as it had been when a beautiful little girl inhabited it, chock full of dolls, toys, and books, a room that spoke of a child who loved being alive and was dearly loved by her parents.

They told me about the school that insisted Shaina had ADHD and needed to be medicated. They told me about how they knew she had no such thing, then they told of how school bullying forced them to accept the diagnosis and drugs because it seemed a less harmful alternative than the ongoing misery at school. They told of the child psychiatrist who put her on an antidepressant because he thought it safer than Ritalin and equally effective in "treating" ADHD. They told me about how he upped her dosage every time the school made renewed complaints about her behavior. They showed me the entry in the *Physicians Desk Reference* where 10 seconds of reading made it clear this 70 lb. girl was being prescribed far too much of the drug. They showed me the sleeping pills and antidepressants this same psychiatrist prescribed to Shaina's mother, without her knowledge or ever having been a patient of his, after disaster struck.

Then they told me how to find her grave.

If ever you are in Smethport visit that graveyard. You might run into the Dunkles; they go there every day, sometimes many times a day, to tend it and read to their daughter. And even if they aren't there Shaina's site is easy to find. The tombstone has her picture on it. There are dolls, wind chimes, pictures, letters and gifts adorning the grave. Only a person with a heart harder than the stones surrounding them wouldn't be moved to tears by it. How did Shaina come to be buried here? Her mother will tell you, in her own words.

DEATH BY DESIPRAMINE: Shaina's Story

My name is Vicky Dunkle and my husband's name is Steve. We live in a small town of about 2000 people. We have a 23-year-old son and a 19-year-old son. We lost our precious 10-year-old daughter, Shaina Louise Dunkle, on February 26, 2001, to desipramine toxicity. She was put on it to treat ADHD. Our daughter would still be alive if we would have followed our hearts instead of the advice of others.

Our lives before the tragedy were like any normal family. We were always on the run between baseball games, football, wrestling, dance class, piano lessons, girl scouts, drill team, and softball games, and lived on hot dogs and pizza night after night. At times we would fit in a walk, ride bikes, swim in the pool, or go to the park and swing. On special family days we went to Darien Lake or Cedar Point. The most important thing was we did it together as a family, and that is what always made it so special. We were very close and did whatever we could for our children. It gave us great pleasure to make them happy.

Shaina was a wonderful child with so much life to give. She could always make you smile and would light up any room by her appearance. She was the center of our world. If her daddy mowed the lawn with the tractor she rode on his lap; if I ran to the store for two seconds she was right there. We would set aside girls days out and go shopping and, of course, never come home without a Barbie or a new outfit. The most important time for me was when we arrived home and would look at each other and say, "Home again, home again, jig-giddy-jig." This is what I miss terribly. Her daddy can't even mow the lawn now because his lap is empty.

When Shaina began school I knew we were going to have problems because she was so close to us and had never been away. Shaina had had a lot of medical difficulties, like two ear surgeries, a reimplantation of her urethra tube, and asthma, so she was used to having her mom and dad and brothers at her beck and call.

The school problems started in kindergarten with the teachers. They would complain that Shaina could not sit for the length of time required, needed to be redirected more than she should have been, was not able to focus, and worried more about other people's business than her own. She was a talker and at school that could be a problem. Shaina was a very spontaneous child and would react and then think.

Well, we made it through the first year of kindergarten. Her teacher said Shaina could go on to first grade but would have some difficulty keeping up, so we decided to repeat kindergarten because I didn't want Shaina to struggle. The second year of kindergarten was much better. Shaina took an immediate liking to her new teacher and actually enjoyed school for the first time and had a much better year. Then she went to first grade and experienced conflicts with this new teacher from day one.

Shaina was excited about going to school at the beginning of the year but slowly went downhill. The teacher she had was not one bit patient or understanding. During this time Shaina would scream and cry, "Please mommy don't make me go to school."

The nightmares began and she would wake up crying. Shaina never did that before. One day she came home in tears and woke up screaming that night. We found out that her teacher had picked up her desk and dumped it on the floor because it was messy. She began to cry when some of the other children laughed at her and was taken out in the hall and scolded because she had cried.

After this episode we decided to home school her. Shaina did her work at day and during the night and was involved in outside activities. She danced jazz, tap, and ballet from the time she was 3 until her death. She took piano lessons, loved to sing, and was involved in Girl Scouts. For second grade we decided to place Shaina back in school. She did fine one-on-one but needed to be with other children her age.

The teacher was wonderful about working with us, nothing like the first-grade teacher. She felt Shaina had learning difficulties and was frustrated because she could not work to her ability, so we took her advice and had Shaina tested for learning disabilities. [2]

She tested in the mildly retarded range and was placed in learning support. Shaina's learning support teachers were absolutely wonderful, she loved them and they loved her. Shaina was Shaina again and enjoyed school.

In March of 1999 I received a letter from the school psychologist requesting that Shaina be evaluated for ADHD by a physician. Shaina was a busy child and a slower learner than others and from time to time became bored easily. She had trouble sitting still and staying on tasks sometimes, but at home was not a problem. From kindergarten until second grade we had refused to medicate Shaina. She had some problems and could be a distraction to others, but she was just like any other child and we knew she would outgrow it. We finally gave in and took her to see a psychiatrist because we found out she was being put out in the hall and isolated from other children again. This is when our nightmare began.

At the first appointment we were pleased with the psychiatrist's manner and rapport with our daughter. He responded well to Shaina and showed genuine concern for her. During that first office visit the psychiatrist drew his conclusion that Shaina had ADHD based on the school psychologist's recommendation. We came out with a prescription for Wellbutrin [bupropion, an antidepressant not related to tricyclic, heterocyclic or SSRI antidepressants; safety and effectiveness in patient below 18 years of age not established].

At the time I didn't really feel any reason to doubt or second-guess the physician. I always felt physicians were next to God, not realizing they are human and can make mistakes just like anyone else. At first Shaina responded well to the medication and her attention and focusing in school showed improvement. But, from time to time school personnel would notify us that Shaina was reverting back so we, in turn, would notify the physician and his choice of action was to increase medication doses.

Shaina began to have constant stomachaches and loss of appetite, so he added Effexor [venlafaxine, a structurally novel antidepressant not related to tricyclic, heterocyclic or SSRI anti-depressants; safety and effectiveness in patient below 18 years of age not established]. Soon I refused to give the Effexor because she couldn't sleep at night and seemed to be very hyper. This is when desipramine [a triclyclic antidepressant; is not recommended for use in children since safety and effectiveness in the pediatric age group have not been established] was introduced into Shaina's life. I had been familiar with Ritalin, Dexedrine, and Adderall being prescribed for ADHD and questioned the physician about why desipramine [3] was a choice. He stated that it is less addictive and has fewer side effects, and that children were known to be crushing and snorting Ritalin.

I had no reason to second-guess or doubt what he was saying to me, and he was the professional, not me. Now I wish I had doubted and second-guessed and even gotten a second or third opinion.

Shaina did well in third grade. She had another wonderful teacher and the support teachers were wonderful, too. Her grades improved, she became more responsible and was able to stay on task and even became a helper to others and would do errands for the teachers, like run the mail and messages. From time to time Shaina would start to slide backward and not be able to con-centrate as well and her grades would slowly go down. When the teachers notified us she was having difficulties we would notify the psychiatrist. Every time he chose to increase medication levels. Shaina began desipramine treatment at 10 mgs a day and by January, 2001, was taking 200 mg daily.

In fourth grade Shaina was having her best year at school ever. Whenever she reverted back to being less attentive and had academic trouble the teachers would notify us and, again, the psychiatrist would increase the medication. In February, 2001, I notified him that Shaina was becoming agitated at school frequently, even throwing a pencil at another student and raising up scissors in her hand at another. This was not like Shaina at all and, of course, we as parents were appalled to even think she would do such a thing. Now we know that such behaviors can be side effects of the desipramine. Neither the psychiatrist nor the pharmacist ever told us about these, or any other problems with the drug.

We noticed that Shaina was putting on weight, with no increase in appetite, and were concerned because she was always thin and fragile. In the shower I noticed she was getting very pudgy and seemed to be hard. But Shaina was always so thin it seemed good to see her putting on weight and beginning to fit into her clothes. Over the weekend I observed Shaina closely for urinating because of her past kidney and urine retention problems and she seemed to be urinating less frequently, which was a concern. But we were going to the psychiatrist the very next day and I felt that he would know what to do. On Monday, February 19, we presented everything that the school and us parents were seeing. The psychiatrist stated that what we were seeing were not side effects and that I was being overly protective. He stated that she was metabolizing the medicine quicker than most and increased the desipramine from 200 mgs to 250 mgs. This was confusing because we were presenting problems, but still he chose to up the prescription, this time by 50 mg instead of 25 mg like before.

On Monday, February 26, I received a phone call from the school nurse at 10 a.m. Shaina had fallen out of her chair in the school library and received a small bump on her right cheek. The nurse stated that she wasn't sure if Shaina may have had a slight seizure, but she appeared to be fine. Shaina's daddy left work to bring her home, and I immediately phoned Shaina's pediatrician. He said to bring her right in. Shaina said she felt fine and wanted to stay home and play Nintendo, but we insisted she be looked at. Shaina brought storybooks and read to us in the car from the time we left until we arrived in his parking lot, which was about 30–35 minutes.

We walked hand-in-hand to the pediatrician's office. When we arrived I took off her coat and wrote her name on the clipboard. When I turned to go sit beside her she began to have a grand mal seizure. I screamed for someone to help me and picked her up in my arms and started to run through the door to the examining room for the doctor. He came around the corner and said, "Vicky, lay Shaina on the floor." I laid her down and placed one arm under her head and kept rubbing her forehead, telling her mommy is here and how much I loved her, "Baby girl, mommy is here and I'm not leaving you." The doctor listened to her heart with a stethoscope and called a code 99. I had worked in a hospital for eleven years as a scrub technician and knew something serious was wrong.

They worked on Shaina for a long time before they finally said she died, but we knew in our hearts she took her last breath while we were there. The horrible thing is that the last thing Shaina saw was my frightened face when I knew I couldn't help her. Steve and I watched helplessly as our daughter died before our eyes and neither one of us could do a thing.

We were drawn up into a world of deceit, lies, and who knows what else. Our whole world was crushed and it has left us to deal with all kinds of doubt, distrust, guilt, hurt, and anger. We now live with the what-ifs. I wish we never trusted and believed in the so-called professionals. If we hadn't believed and trusted and just followed our hearts, not the advice of others, our precious Shaina would be alive now and we would not be telling this story.

Shaina Dunkle was our world and our world was crushed. The sunshine left and the darkness appeared; our lives are sad, empty, and lonely. They say each day gets better, but believe us, it doesn't get any better; you learn to tolerate life, but it doesn't get any better. We now visit our child in a cemetery 2 to 3 times a day while others continue to live their lives and children ride their bikes and go on like nothing has happened.

I found out that desipramine is a tricyclic antidepressant that is not FDA approved for children because its safety and effectiveness for children have not been proven. Physicians continue to prescribe "off label" medications like these that are not safe. For people who get an overdose of desipramine there is no antidote to counteract it, they die. Side effects are not properly discussed and you are told what they want you to know, not what you need to know. If for one minute we had been told the proper side effects of desipramine, Shaina would never have taken one dose. Desipramine is the most toxic antidepressant of any of the tricyclic medications. There have been at least seven deaths associated with desipramine use in normal, healthy children. They die suddenly, with no warning, within minutes. [4]

To all the parents who are struggling with, "Is my child ADHD and should we medicate or not medicate?" all I can say is that one day we were where you maybe are now, and if we could only go back and do things differently we sure would. There is no way we would ever have put our daughter on medicine. I stress very strongly to follow your heart and not the advice of others. If you do choose to follow advice, then check, double check, and triple check before you make a decision.

We now live with the heartbreak of wondering if our precious Shaina knows we never wanted this to happen. All we wanted is for her to fit in with the other kids and be like they were so she would fit into society and be accepted. Shaina fit into our world just fine, and we loved and accepted her for who she was.

* * *

Shaina Dunkle and her family were failed by professionals who should have known better every step of the way, from teacher to psychologist to psychiatrist, and plenty of other professionals who abused the trust placed in them, whose cumulative actions led to the death of a wonderful little girl who was perfectly normal. But wasn't her academic performance behind the norm? Didn't she have trouble staying focused in class? Yes, and these were normal variations that occur within a population of children, not diseases. Children develop at different rates; some are better or worse at certain things than others; some children can sit still all day, while others want to be in motion; some children learn well within school's confines, others are active learners who do not experience success or satisfaction behind a desk. Why not embrace them all, instead of embracing the ones who easily fit into the predominant educational system and declaring the ones who need something else to be damaged goods?

In Shaina's case the trouble began with the notion that lower than average academic performance was evidence of a learning disability. If you look at a textbook on learning disabilities you will probably find a statement inside claiming that learning disabilities are the result of some kind of impairment to the central nervous system (brain damage). As with ADHD absolutely no scientific evidence of this has ever been found—it is entirely assumed based on "discrepancy" testing that supposedly reveals a child's performance in, say, reading or math to be less than what is expected, just as ADHD is assumed if attention span is less than expected.

In Shaina's case, something that has happened to millions of other children, too, the step from diagnosing a learning disability to "discovering" ADHD is a small one. And if Shaina hadn't died the diagnoses could easily have continued on, to include bipolar, anxiety, or a multitude of other things, as has also happened to a rapidly escalating number of children.

How can one disorder be piled on top of another? How can one medication be supplemented by a revolving door of others, forming a toxic stew nobody can predict the risks of? The core reason is the deliberate confusion between what is a verifiable disease and that warrants treatment and what is not. Before proceeding any further let us make clear the obvious fact that there are plenty of things children suffer from, like neglect and abuse, and plenty of bad living situations they inhabit that cause just as much, and sometimes more, misery than a disease. To be free of disease does not mean one is free from suffering. The distinction is that a medical disease (with abnormality=disease, with the abnormality needing treatment to be made normal or more nearly normal) may call for medical intervention, i.e., surgery or drugs. Something that is not a medical disease, like living in a dysfunctional family or attending a school that is a poor fit, requires an intervention that is not medical, which means counseling, a change in circumstances, or anything else that can be done to best meet a child's real needs. What it does not mean are diagnoses of mental "diseases" and the prescription of dangerous drugs.

WHAT IS A DISEASE?

Before we go any further in our discussion of ADHD we need to examine the meaning of the word "disease" and the means physicians use to diagnose diseases. The misuse and perversion of powerful medical terms such as "disease," "syndrome," and "pathology" are at the heart of the promotion of ADHD. Unless we understand the basic principles of how medical science determines what constitutes disease, we are doomed to being misled by those who weave illusions of disease for profit.

Stedman's Medical Dictionary, 25th Edition, [5] defines disease as the following:

> *Disease: 1. Morbus; illness; sickness; an interruption, cessation, or disorder of bodily functions, systems or organs. 2. A morbid entity characterized usually by at least two of these*

criteria: recognized etiologic * agent(s), identifiable groups of signs and symptoms, or consistent anatomical alterations. See also syndrome.

* Origin, Cause

In fact, in the ethical practice of medicine the definition of "disease" is much more simple and straightforward—disease = abnormality. There do not even need to be symptoms, which are complaints brought to a physician that are wholly subjective. For example, a person with no complaints/symptoms may be found on chest x-ray to have a spot on the lung which, in turn, may be found by surgery and biopsy to be lung cancer. Similarly, most cancers have no known cause. Most cases of diabetes and of epilepsy (seizures) have no known or discernible cause or etiology either, making the cancer, diabetes and epilepsy no less abnormalities and no less diseases. Consider Lou Gehrig's disease, amyotrophic lateral sclerosis, no less a disease, no less a uniformly fatal disease, despite the fact that it's etiology (cause) is not known.

Whether or not a patient complains of symptoms, whether or not the cause is known, real diseases all have this is common—an objective abnormality is demonstrable; the abnormality is the disease.

Thus, no matter how lengthy various medical dictionary definitions may be or how much fudging gets done by those who would invent "diseases" for profit, when you get down to it, disease = abnormality. No disease = disease-free = no abnormality = normal. An important point here is that our bodies (including the brain) are presumed to be normal, just as we presume individuals to be innocent, until proven otherwise. When investigating the possibility of disease or guilt, the tests must be rigorous and the results must be clear. Then, and only then, can meaningful intervention take place. Without the assumption that we are normal or innocent, until clear, reliable, objective evidence tells us differently, we are wide open to wrongful diagnoses and wrongful convictions. In both cases, as we saw in the example of Shaina Dunkle, the unnecessary suffering that follows can be tragic.

Always be aware of how badly language and science are per-
verted in descriptions of ADHD. The term "disease" is avoided
because there is no proof ADHD is one and writers on the topic do
not want to raise alarms with the use of the term. Whenever ADHD
is spoken of as being a chemical imbalance, disorder, syndrome, or
any other term that denotes a disruption of normal functioning
that has biological roots, it is disease that is really being spoken
of. But talk is cheap. The ADHD promoters can go on all they
want about suspicions of neurological impairments or a genetic in-
heritance: they could blame the Great Pumpkin, too, which would
have equal credibility.

Medical diagnoses cannot be made by opinion, suspicion, or
committee; there must be proven facts, a demonstrated, demonstrable abnormality. If there are no abnormalities the result is
exactly what we have now, a perversion of language and ethics so
twisted that any normal person can be labeled as suffering from
a disease.

A physician's first duty to every patient is not to determine
which disease they have, but, more fundamentally, to determine
whether or not they have any disease at all. Even though patients
present to doctors with complaints, or symptoms, as many as half
of all patients seeing family or general practitioners are found to
be free of disease. By process of elimination, their symptoms are
determined to be due to the stress of everyday living and include
psychological and psychiatric symptoms, and ailments such as
depression, anxiety, panic, insomnia, and so on. These patients
require an understanding, compassionate explanation of the nature of their symptoms and how the stress of everyday life can be
overwhelming at times. Assured that they have no actual disease,
the patient is then better equipped to cope and make necessary ad-
justments, which may include behavioral therapy or counseling.

The duty and responsibility of diagnosis, of determining
whether or not disease is present and, if so, what disease, resides with
the physician, not with the patient, parent, teacher, psychologist, or
social worker. The physician is the one with the specialized medi-

cal training and experience that are critical to making distinctions between what are diseases and what are not diseases. Without the proper training and experience no such competence can exist.

As we will soon see below, psychiatrists, though trained as physicians, have gotten into the habit of making disease diagnoses without following the proper protocol. And, sad to say, this is a trend that family practitioners and pediatricians, along with many other specialists, have been fueling with their own diagnoses of ADHD and other similarly non-existent conditions.

Physicians often encounter new patients who have moved to their areas of practice from somewhere else. In such cases the physician assuming responsibility would be foolish and put herself at legal risk if she did not verify that, 1) any diagnosis the patient came with was correct and, 2) the ongoing treatment was appropriate, beneficial and free of deleterious side effects. Regardless of who the referring physician or medical facility has been, I (senior author, Fred Baughman, MD) always take steps to verify the diagnosis. In more than a few instances I have found the diagnosis to be wrong, or found no organic disease at all.

Alarmingly, the majority of physicians, mostly psychiatrists, family practitioners, pediatricians, and neurologists, faced with a given diagnosis of ADHD, usually provided or initiated by school personnel who are totally unqualified to do so, accept it, along with all the unverified claims that it is an actual disease, something wrong with the brain of the child. The prescription for Adderall, Ritalin, or one of the other ADHD medications is provided automatically, as if by reflex. Medicine should never be practiced this way. If the physician has found no evidence of disease, that must be said. Nothing less is owed the patient.

I have had patients and parents of patients tell me they are certain, having read articles or books, that they or their children have ADHD. Others come to me convinced their children have it because a teacher, a school counselor, or psychologist said so. I have also had teachers tell me that if I do not provide the coveted ADHD diagnosis for a particular child they have targeted that they will refer the family to somebody else who will. The physician's responsibility is clear—they must resist this pressure and conduct an unbiased evaluation. Those who knowingly attach unwarranted disease designations or diagnoses for purposes of financial gain are anti-Hippocratic (the oath to "First do no harm"), anti-scientific, and reprehensible.

Before I even begin my assessment of a new patient I explain my duty of diagnosis to the patient. Then, with their permission, I proceed to take a thorough history, which is the most important aspect of diagnosis and one that usually consumes more time than the examination to follow.

Next is the physical examination, where the physician may or may not elicit telling signs in the course of it. Maybe he will see a rash, hear a heart murmur, feel a lump in a breast, or smell a distinctive odor about the patient with late-stage liver disease. These are signs and are objective. By contrast, symptoms are complaints elicited from the patient, or parents on behalf of a child, and are subjective. Therefore, it is no surprise that so many turn out not to have abnormalities or diseases. This does not mean the presenting complaints are contrived. Often these symptoms are real physical manifestations of stress, like sleeplessness, loss of appetite, pain, or anxiety, and an explanation that the patient does not have a disease should be reassuring, especially when they can be directed to the appropriate treatment, such as problem-directed talk therapy.

If, on the other hand, I find consistent symptoms plus abnormal signs on examination, I am justified in concluding that some disease, yet to be determined, is present. Only the finding of a definite abnormality (an objective sign) allows for the conclusion that a disease is present. The doctor's next duty, separate from the first step, is to proceed with differential diagnosis, that is, to determine what disease, from a list of possible diseases, the patient might have, like diabetes, congestive heart failure, or cancer, for example.

At this point blood and urine tests, x-rays, scans, amino acid chromatography [6], or any of numerous other procedures may be ordered. In diabetes the blood sugar would be elevated and sugar found in the urine as well. In kidney disease the blood urea nitrogen (BUN) would be elevated, proof that urea, a breakdown product poisonous to the body, was not being normally excreted. Had the patient a one-sided epileptic seizure leading to a suspicion of brain tumor a CT (Computed Tomography) or MRI (Magnetic Resonance Imaging) scan could be done to confirm the diagnosis.

I reiterate that a disease or a medical syndrome must have a physical or chemical abnormality or it is not a disease (or a medical syndrome or anything physical or biologic). A physician may suspect the existence of a disease, but before she can diagnose it, that is, say conclusively that one is present, she must demonstrate an abnormality by some means at her disposal.

For a disease to exist, pathology, a word denoting an abnormality, must be present. This abnormality may be obvious, as in the case of a benign or cancerous tumor that can be felt by palpating the belly wall. Or it may not be palpable or even visible to the surgeon's eye, but recognizable as cancerous and abnormal only when a piece of the tissue or a Pap smear showing malignant cells is viewed under a microscope.

Some diseases are only recognized by the characteristic alteration of the body's chemistry that they cause. In phenylketonuria a defective gene leads to an absence of the enzyme phenylalanine hydroxylase and to phenylpyruvic acid in the urine and mental retardation. In galactosemia a defective gene leads to the absence of an enzyme needed to convert the sugar, galactose, to gluscose, resulting in malnutrition, liver enlargement, cataracts, retardation and death. In Hunter's and Hurler's syndromes, genetic forms of gargoylism, complex chemicals called mucopolysaccharides, accumulate in the tissues and urine and result in death. Wilson's disease, cystinosis, citrullinuria, fructosuria, Gaucher's disease, Hartnup's disease, homocystinuria, porphyria, and many, many more are real genetic diseases causing real chemical imbalances at the same time.

In all of these real "inborn errors of metabolism" caused by defective genes there are, in addition to the chemical abnormalities, clear gross and microscopic abnormalities of the brain and, in most such diseases, of virtually all of the organ systems and tissues of the body. Even diabetics have gross and microscopic abnormalities of blood vessels and most organs.

All of these medical principles have a direct bearing on the evaluation of ADHD. That ADD was "discovered" (actually voted into existence by a committee) over twenty years ago and is still without a confirmatory, characteristic, abnormality anywhere in the brain or body is, if nothing else, reason for suspicion. If ADD/ADHD was solely meant as a shorthand means of describing a particular set of behaviors the terms would be less unsavory (though "disorder" would have to be removed), but for it to be presented as a chemical imbalance, genetic defect, neurological abnormality, disorder (which means something is abnormal and therefore a disease is present) is in direct conflict with the legitimate, scientific, ethical practice of medicine. ADHD is not a medical reality in any sense. To represent it as one is fraud.

Sometimes the argument is advanced that ADHD is no less a disease than diabetes because both share the lack of a known etiology (cause). Such statements are meant to mislead. Many real diseases, characterized by real, distinctive abnormalities (pathology), are without a known cause or etiology. The many physical and chemical abnormalities in diabetes make it a disease. Diabetics have a diminished number of beta cells in the pancreas, secreting below-normal levels of insulin, leaving blood sugar and urine sugar levels abnormally high. We speak of its pathology and pathogenesis (the development and evolution of a disease throughout its entire course) even though we do not know the cause of the diminished number of beta cells. It was also obvious that AIDS was a real disease, a catastrophic one, long before the discovery of its etiology, the HIV virus.

ADHD, on the other hand, has no measurable physical or chemical abnormalities. This makes it a theory in search of validation. It does not matter how many studies of ADHD are done, research papers written, money spent, or years looking for evidence. Without identifying an abnormality ADHD can never rise above the level of speculation or fraud. Legitimate scientific speculation it is not.

Another favored strategy of those who invent diseases like ADHD is to write of the pathology of it, even using "Pathology" as a title, as though one had been proven, i.e., a physical or chemical abnormality, and then commence a discussion of current hypotheses while saying nothing concrete about pathology or abnormalities. Terms are regularly thrown out, like "pathogenesis," "psychopathology," "neuropsychiatry," or "neurobiology," attempting to convey that things physical, biological and "diseased" are present, when in fact no such thing has been proved.

In AIDS we have an example of how, in medicine, we often interchange the terms "disease" and "syndrome." Both terms denote the presence of a consistent physical or chemical abnormality that can be diagnosed. Those who invent false diseases are inclined to embrace the terms "syndrome" and "disorder" rather than "disease" because they suspect, correctly, no doubt, that these are less likely to provoke objections. In keeping with this the last letter of ADHD stands for disorder, not disease, because the term is viewed as providing more latitude. Adding to the confusion, the term "syndrome" has been regularly bandied about in sociology, psychology, and psychiatry (prior to the days of biopsychiatry) and is meant to denote a combination of behaviors without assuming the presence of physical or chemical abnormalities.

When ADHD or any other psychiatric creation is presented as having a medical basis, however, as is the norm today, then the medical language employed must remain true to its real meaning. So, when a medical diagnosis of ADHD is made, we are being told that the disorder is present because of an abnormality that exists within the child or adult being diagnosed, which means, in medicine, that a disease is present. And if we are told that ADHD is a neurological syndrome or chemical imbalance, it means the same, that an abnormality exists and therefore a disease is present. Put simply, as mentioned above, disorder = syndrome = pathology = abnormality = disease. With ADHD, however, no abnormality is ever identified with any of the legitimate means at medicine's disposal. When a doctor, trained in the principles of medical diagnosis outlined here, presents ADHD as a disease, no matter the equivalent term that gets used, it is not the ethical practice of medicine; it is the practice of deceit. It is 100% fraud.

HOW A REAL DISEASE IS DISCOVERED AND VERIFIED

I have over 35 years experience as a front-line adult and pediatric neurologist. In addition to maintaining a full time practice I also conducted research and discovered and verified real diseases. In order to make any kind of legitimate medical diagnosis, evidence that meets proper scientific standards must exist, something that has yet to happen for a single diagnosis of ADHD.

As I explained above, symptoms or complaints alone do not a disease or diagnosis make. Sooner or later a physical abnormality must be demonstrated. All physicians, including psychiatrists so long as they count themselves as members of the medical profession, have as their primary duty to determine if a real disease, confirmed (by physical exam, x-ray, scan, blood, urine, or spinal fluid test, etc.) by a physical abnormality is present or not present.

The secondary duty of physicians, that of disclosure and informed consent, is to lay out, in understandable terms to the patient or parent, the particulars about their condition—whether they have an abnormality/disease or not; how it will behave with no treatment and how the treatment or prescription proposed will beneficially alter the outcome. If the disease is untreatable that, too, comes under the heading of disclosure and informed consent.

It is also the duty of physicians to inform patients when they do not have a real disease and direct them to the proper alternatives for treatment (non-medical). Patients with chronic fatigue, headache, stomachache, insomnia, etc. in whom repeated examinations fail to reveal a physical or chemical abnormality are likely to have, by process of elimination, a psychogenic, i.e., stress-induced disorder. Many such patients and their physicians and health care providers who profit from it believe they have a life-long "manageable" disorder and refuse to accept the diagnosis of "no organic disease." For these patients, symptom management can go on indefinitely, making them "profit centers" in perpetuity who may never be cured. If, however, they have a capable, ethical, scientific physician, the road to a cure and a normal life can be paved by a proper, educated, approach to their problem.

Just because a presenting problem does not meet the criteria for a disease does not mean the suffering endured is therefore trivial or the treatment unimportant. A person going through life with constant headaches, insomnia, or unyielding fatigue, just to name a few, may well experience greater distress that somebody with a diagnosed disease, which is all the more reason to address it properly. To make a medical diagnosis and prescribe medical treatment for a non-medical issue only piles more problems on somebody already struggling with a heavy load.

Now let us look at how real diseases are discovered and verified. During the time I practiced in Grand Rapids a 23 month-old girl was brought to me who, like two of her nine siblings, was slow to walk and unsteady afoot. As for the first question, is there a disease or not? The answer was clearly "yes." Her problem presented constantly and, accompanied by a delayed onset of walking, was a definite abnormality, signifying the presence of real disease, in this instance most likely of the cerebellum, the part of the brain having to do with balance and locomotion. With three of nine siblings and no other relatives involved, there was every reason to believe that their disease was due to an autosomal recessive genetic disorder, but I wasn't sure which of the cerebellar diseases or ataxias (incoordination afoot) it was. No tumor or conspicuous wasting was seen on the brain scan. It had to be something qualitatively, functionally wrong with the cerebellum.

I showed movies of the affected children to groups of neurologists. All agreed that they had a cerebellar disease but none could identify it further. It was only with the passage of years and the appearance of spider-like veins on their eyes, face, and ears that the diagnosis of ataxia-telangiectasia, or Louis-Bar Syndrome [7], the only such case in my 33 years of practice, was diagnosed. Although the presence of a definite, real disease had been determined the first day the children were seen, just which of the many cerebellar diseases the children had awaited the emergence of further signs some years later. But this was not the only disease they had. There was a second genetic disease, one that had not been discovered yet!

The 23-month-old girl, a brother, their mother, two maternal aunts, and a maternal uncle had curly hair, fused eyelids at birth (needing surgical separation), and finger and toe-nail dysplasia (which means ridged and gnarled), the combination of which I described as CHANDS [8] (curly hair, ankyloblepharon, nail dysplasia syndrome) and, after my original conjectures and further review with colleagues a few years later, concluded it was an autosomal recessive trait, [9] like Louis-Bar Syndrome.

Here I began with a little girl initially brought to me to see why she walked poorly and late and I, the physician, determined that there were not one but two real diseases present—one extremely rare and the other never before discovered or described but which could be pinned down by very specific objective signs. Despite years of trying, ADHD has never been discovered, which means it is impossible to provide a medical description of it.

Because the abnormalities of CHANDS are relatively harmless, there is justification for calling it a syndrome. Those seeking to confuse the issue often refer to ADHD as a syndrome, a neurological syndrome, hoping to glide over the diagnostic pitfalls by avoiding the more worry-inducing label of "disease." But, medically and biologically speaking, both terms refer to a distinctive condition with a detectable physical or chemical abnormality. ADHD has never met this standard.

THE MAKING OF PSYCHOPHARMACOLOGY: HOW MONEY FUELS THE INVASION OF PSYCHIATRY INTO DAILY LIFE

For 10 of the 11 years that I (senior author Fred Baughman, MD) practiced in Grand Rapids, Michigan, I shared an office and a fruitful collaboration with Dr. Robert Troske, a perceptive, humane psychiatrist. Bob had patients, including the many I referred to him, whose problems were not organic (no disease) but psychogenic (of a psychological nature, no disease). He helped them to better understand themselves, their stresses and symptoms, and to better cope with their difficulties. He used psychotropic medications, but sparingly, as an adjunct to treatment and not as the treatment itself. Never did he demean and dehumanize his patients by failing to communicate with them or by drugging them one-dimensionally, as if it were possible to treat their brains like bags of neurotransmitters awaiting chemical manipulation.

Another thing about Bob was his "nose" for things organic, meaning having a sense that a disease might present and that a physical examination was called for. At times patients were referred to him that he suspected had something other than a mental or psychiatric problem. It is not that he knew exactly what organic disease they had but, more fundamentally, he understood the disease/no disease concept and often sensed correctly when disease was present. He would then refer the patient back to the referring physician or to me for further clarification of the diagnosis. The others, struggling, troubled human beings were his patients and he respected them and helped them cope and overcome, concepts lost on present day biopsychiatrists seduced by the anti-scientific, for profit, disease/drug model.

By the early 80s there was a mounting glut of physicians in general and psychiatrists in particular. As we will see, that glut pushed the development of new diagnoses, a market expansion to accommodate both the growing workforce of psychiatrists and the desire of drug companies to make money. Gaining force through the 80s and 90s was the increasing proclivity of psychiatrists to employ one-dimensional drugging for just about any problem a patient came to them with. Claiming time efficiency, these psychiatrists deigned to look into the nature of their patients' problems or to credit them with intelligence or humanity. What was important was to identify the chemical imbalance, prescribe the balancer, a pill, then use the DSM codes to bill for services.

I have often pointed out to my psychiatrist colleagues who are given to waxing biologic that they do not do general physical examinations, or neurological examinations, or laboratory, x-ray, or scanning diagnostics. How, then, can they possibly claim to demonstrate organic, biologic, or chemical abnormalities, the very things necessary to diagnose actual diseases? But diagnose they do, in violation of the most basic precepts they learned in medical school.

During the mid-80s, my having moved to California in 1975, I increasingly found psychiatrists doing this with the patients I sent them and disapproved. I stopped sending my patients to psychiatrists and began referring them to psychologists, family counselors, and social workers, professionals without a disease orientation or prescribing privileges, who were more likely to provide humane counseling, rather than simply drugging patients and sending them back out the door.

The role of psychiatry was defined in 1948 when neuropsychiatry was divided into two specialties. One was neurology, dealing with organic/physical diseases of the brain. The other was psychiatry, which addressed emotional and behavioral conditions in normal human beings after all possible physical diseases had been ruled out.[10]

There was, therefore, no such thing as a psychiatric disease then, and there is not today, either.

With the advent of psychiatric drugs in the 1950s psychiatry's reach began to expand dramatically, eventually achieving its current state where territory is claimed within almost all areas of life. As more drugs became available and accepted for use outside of the limited population of the severely disturbed, the number of possible psychiatric diagnoses grew. In 1953 the DSM listed 112 disorders, then 163 in 1968, 224 in 1980, and 374 in 1994. Ready to medicalize all aspects of life, the DSM extends itself to the point of absurdity, even willing to diagnose a child with a distaste for math as having developmental-arithmetic disorder—"dyscalculia." (Now there's something that doesn't add up.)

The reach of psychiatry into aspects of normal life may seem incredible to those unfamiliar with it. But a current example of one disease now being formulated is illuminating. In a recent development, psychiatry, for the first time, is seeking to diagnose couples or groups of people, rather than limiting itself to individuals. How is that done? With relational disorders. These will label squabbling couples or fighting families as being afflicted with a mental illness (disease) that is evidenced by difficulty getting along with each other. Sure, people in all kinds of social arrangements have trouble getting along, but should that fact become medicalized? As silly as it sounds (and it has not been accepted yet), bear in mind the purpose of making life's difficulties into official disorders. By giving them a name and a numeric code to put in a box on an insurance form, an increased population of potential patients is opened up with the possibility of making money on them. The DSM is generally referred to as the "psychiatric bible" because of all the disorders and their descriptions it contains. A more accurate term is "billing bible," as having a numeric code to write in on an insurance form increases the chances of getting paid for treating it.

As medical research has developed over time the rate of new disease discovery has dropped and fewer and fewer remain undetected. Yet, now psychiatry comes along attaching the label of disease to things that apply to millions of people. What could be more widespread that arguing with your spouse? You can't make money off a disease that only a few people have, but when the prevalence goes up so does the profitability—hence, the "discovery" of things like ADHD and relational disorders whose symptoms mirror normal human behaviors.

Because proof for the claimed psychiatric disorders is not required, they are able to go further and further afield in the search for new billing opportunities. All that is needed to justify another one is a new set of symptoms, which are always subjective, and can be voted into existence by a committee.

As the United States Congress Office of Technology [11] put it, "Research has yet to identify specific biological causes for any of these disorders. Mental disorders are classified on the basis of symptoms because there are as yet no biological markers or laboratory tests for them." Yet, psychiatry, over the years, has come to insist more and more strenuously that these disorders do have a biological basis, then, without any evidence of such, seeks to describe them as legitimate medical conditions. Thomas Szasz, an emeritus professor of psychiatry at Syracuse University, explains, "The designation disease can only be justified when the cause can be related to a demonstrated anatomical lesion, infection, or some other physiological defect. As there is no such evidence for any mental disorder, the term disease is a misnomer; in fact, it is fraudulent."

What psychiatry has descended to, with physicians in plenty of other specialties following their lead, is the abandonment of their scientific concept of disease. Why? In order to make room for a much broader definition of disease which, in practice, is anything that third-party payers (insurance companies) will foot the bill for. This means that the creative invention and marketing (and we've all seen the advertisements that flood our television screens, radio airwaves, newspapers, magazines, and internet servers) of illusory diseases that afflict the largest possible number become paramount in an environment where swaying opinions count more heavily than scientific results—and pay better, too.

The Hippocratic Oath is being eclipsed by hypocrisy. When the other, non-psychiatric faculty members of the nations medical schools, say nothing of this fraud and poisoning, they are accomplices.

Chapter Five

THE DSM: DANGEROUSLY STRANGE MANEUVERS

We do not have an independent, valid test for ADHD, and there are no data to indicate that ADHD is due to a brain malfunction.

- Final statement of the panel from the National Institutes of Health Consensus Conference on ADHD, November 18, 1998

Near the end of the 17th century Jonathan Swift published a satiric piece called *A Modest Proposal.* In it he advocated breeding children as food in order to feed adults, thereby eliminating food shortages. Readers were horrified that anybody, satire or not, would dare raise the subject. Today, though we have not reached the point where broiled kids are served up for dinner, millions of defenseless children around the world are being ravaged by a predatory frenzy, and the sections of the DSM-IV that deal with psychiatric disorders in children serve as instructional manuals for branding them so that meal time can begin. And who are those at the trough?

When we look at the diagnostic criteria for ADHD in the DSM-IV [1] [2] it almost looks like somebody wrote it in jest, as though Jonathan Swift had been reincarnated in order to lampoon psychiatry's diagnostic process. Surely the individual responsible will step forward someday and admit that the whole thing was a joke, and that he never dreamed it would be taken seriously, and that he is very sorry for the whole mess, right? After all, what could be more absurd than a guide for tagging children as mentally ill simply because they act like children? The unfortunate truth is that it is taken seriously, and the consequences for those it is used against are not funny.

Just as bad as pegging normal children with imaginary disorders is the step that comes next—using the diagnosis as an excuse for forcing normal children to take powerful drugs in order to control unwanted behaviors, like fidgeting, not following directions, doing sloppy work, getting out of a chair, or even daydreaming. Maybe diagnosing and drugging children are not as bad as eating them, but both are predatory practices conducted at the expense of children whose interests are sacrificed.

Below we begin with the DSM IV's guidelines for diagnosing ADHD. Following that we will look at how, based on their success, the same process is being used to label them with a swelling number of afflictions, from anxiety to bi-polar disorders. As you read the ADHD criteria try to a imagine a child who *does not* exhibit enough of the behaviors listed to qualify for a diagnosis, especially if these incredibly subjective standards are being applied by somebody predisposed to find them. As fathers we would be inclined to worry about a child who did *not* behave this way. It should not take long before you understand why Dr. William Carey said, in his presentation to the NIH Consensus Conference, "Common assumptions about ADHD include that it is clearly distinguishable from normal behavior, constitutes a neurodevelopmental disability, is relatively uninfluenced by the environment...All of these assumptions must be challenged because of the weakness of empirical support and the strength of contrary evidence."

Diagnostic criteria for Attention–Deficit/ Hyperactivity Disorder

A. Either (1) or (2):

(1) six (or more) of the following symptoms of **inattention** have persisted for at least 6 months to a degree that is maladaptive and inconsistent with developmental level:

Inattention

(a) often fails to give close attention to details or makes careless mistakes in schoolwork, work, or other activities

(b) often has difficulty sustaining attention in tasks or play activities

(c) often does not seem to listen when spoken to directly

(d) often does not follow through on instructions and fails to finish schoolwork, chores, or duties in the workplace (not due to oppositional behavior or failure to understand instructions).

(e) often has difficulty organizing tasks and activities

(f) often avoids, dislikes, or is reluctant to engage in tasks that require sustained mental effort (such as schoolwork or homework)

(g) often loses things necessary for tasks or activities (e.g., toys, school assignments, pencils, books, or tools)

(h) is often distracted by extraneous stimuli

(i) is often forgetful in daily activities

(2) six (or more) of the following symptoms of **hyperactivity-impulsivity** have persisted for at least 6 months to a degree that is maladaptive and inconsistent with developmental level:

Hyperactivity

(a) often fidgets with hands or feet or squirms in seat

(b) often leaves seat in classroom or in other situations in which remaining seated is expected

(c) often runs about or climbs excessively in situations in which it is inappropriate (in adolescents or adults, may be limited to subjective feelings of restlessness)

(d) often has difficulty playing or engaging in leisure activities quietly

(e) is often "on the go" or often acts as if "driven by a motor"

(f) often talks excessively

Impulsivity

(g) often blurts out answers before questions have been completed

(h) often has difficulty awaiting turn

(i) often interrupts or intrudes on others (e.g., butts into conversations or games)

B. Some hyperactive-impulsive or inattentive symptoms that caused impairment were present before age 7 years.

C. Some impairment from the symptoms is present in two or more settings (e.g., at school [or work] and at home).

D. There must be clear evidence of clinically significant impairment in social, academic, or occupational functioning.

E. The symptoms do not occur exclusively during the course of a Pervasive Developmental Disorder, Schizophrenia, or other Psychotic Disorder and are not better accounted for by another mental disorder (e.g., Mood Disorder, Anxiety Disorder, Dissociative Disorder, or a Personality Disorder).

The first few sentences of the diagnostic features portion of the DSM IV section on ADHD states:

> *The essential feature of Attention-Deficit/Hyperactivity Disorder is a persistent pattern of inattention and/or hyperactivity-impulsivity that is more frequently displayed and more severe than is typically observed in individuals at a comparable level of development (Criterion A). Some hyperactive-impulsive or inattentive symptoms that cause impairment must have been present before age 7 years, although many individuals are diagnosed after the symptoms have been present for a number of years, especially in the case of individuals with the Predominantly Inattentive Type (Criterion B). Some impairment from the symptoms must be present in at least two settings (e.g., at home and at school or work)(Criterion C). There must be clear evidence of interference with developmentally appropriate social, academic, or occupational functioning (Criterion D).*

Right from the beginning there are serious shortcomings that illustrate why the ADHD diagnostic criteria are so open to misuse and abuse, even apart from the fact that there is no scientific basis. The first sentence states, "The essential feature of Attention-Deficit/Hyperactivity Disorder is a persistent pattern of inattention and/or hyperactivity-impulsivity that is more frequently displayed and more severe than is typically in individuals at a comparable level of development (Criterion A)." At what point does a pattern of inattention and hyperactivity-impulsivity become persistent? Do the patterns always have to be the same? Is occasionally similar enough? How often do these have to be seen in order to be considered frequent, every day, twice an hour, three times per month? And how much worse do they have to be in order to qualify as more severe than typical? What, exactly, is typical anyway? Typical for a classroom, a school district, the county, country, or world?

When it comes to development, anybody who has paid attention to children knows they develop at different rates, with some
capacities coming "online" earlier or later than others, with different children having different areas of strength or weakness. With
so much going on in developmental terms, how do you compare
one child's package of developing attributes to another child's, or
group of children, let alone decide what is normal or not? Sure,
in extreme cases it is possible to say that a child's development is
lagging so far behind the norm for a particular age that there is
cause for concern, but in the majority of cases the variations are
well within the normal range.

As for hyperactive, impulsive, or inattentive symptoms being present before age 7, it is difficult to find a pre-7 year old who
does not display these frequently. Bear in mind, too, that half of
all pre-7 year olds will be more active, impulsive, and inattentive than the average, so at what point does it become a problem?
Further, no mention is made of the kinds of environments kids
are functioning in. A child with active, involved parents who are
tolerant of childhood behaviors and encourage her to explore is
far less likely to be considered hyperactive or impulsive than a
child with sedentary parents for whom keeping up is difficult,
especially if they are not tolerant of the things they cannot keep
up with. The parent who is interested in a variety of activities and
has the ability to juggle many of them at once is much less likely
to see a child with a short attention span as a problem than the
parent who insists on strict order and completing each task in
sequence before starting on anything else.

The same holds for observers of children who make judgments about the ADHD criteria, judgments that will be influenced
by their own lifestyles, values, education, and professional pref-
erences. In the case of educators, they know their observations
will have a lot to do with whether or not a child is diagnosed and
medicated. If getting the child put on a drug that will make him
easier to manage is a possible outcome of the evaluation process,
then it is easy to see how the criteria can be misapplied, even by

people who truly believe they are acting in the child's best interest (which does not excuse their bad judgment or the harm done to children as a result).

Maybe you can find yourself described in some of what follows in the DSM, as both authors of this book have:

Individuals with this disorder may fail to give close attention to details or may make careless mistakes in schoolwork or other tasks (Criterion A1a). Work is often messy and performed carelessly and without considered thought. Individuals often have difficulty sustaining attention in tasks or play activities and often find it hard to persist with tasks until completion. (Criterion A1b). They often appear as if their mind is elsewhere or is if they are not listening or did not hear what has just been said (Criterion A1c). There may be frequent shifts from one uncompleted activity to another. Individuals diagnosed with this disorder may begin a task, move on to another, then turn to yet something else, prior to completing any one task. They often do not follow through on requests or instructions and fail to complete schoolwork, chores, or other duties.

Does that sound like anybody you know? If not yourself, then you certainly have come across many adults this fits, and for children it is common and perfectly normal. How do we define what not giving close attention to details is? Does it mean we can't, have some trouble with it, or are bored, disinterested, or simply determined not to go along? Are there other details that are paid attention to? And what about levels of interest? If you are doing something that captivates you and is a good fit with your talents, then you naturally pay closer attention to details. If, however, you are bored, doing something you do not like, or champing at the bit to finish a task you are uninterested in order to move on to something more alluring, then details are not going to get your best attention. As for careless mistakes, is that because of boredom or lack of interest, maybe a form of resistance to a task you resent having to perform, or maybe just an indication that it is not an area of strength for you?

The DSM continues to make matters worse, saying a bit further on:

> *Tasks that require sustained mental effort are experienced as unpleasant and markedly aversive. As a result, these individuals typically avoid or have a strong dislike for activities that demand sustained self-application and mental effort or that require organizational demands or close concentration (e.g., homework or paperwork) (Criterion A1f).*

This section is biased against people of a more active, physical bent, which many children are simply because of the age they are at. If you derive the most satisfaction from activities and occupations that allow you to involve your body to a high degree and find sitting still in a chair doing dull pen, paper, and computer tasks to be unpleasant, then you might have ADHD, according to this. In schools this covers the kids, especially boys again, who find school requirements dull (which they often are) and unrewarding. Of course a person is going to have an aversion to tasks they do not like or find at odds with their nature, interests, and abilities. In schools, then, educators have a ideal mechanism for targeting children who resist going along with the educational methods and curriculum the school is determined to force on them, one way or another.

As adults we gravitate toward careers and environments that match up with our likes, talents, and capacities. Children required to go to school have not had that opportunity yet and are at risk of being considered neurologically abnormal simply because they are at the mercy of inept educators who are disturbed when they do not "fit" well in a traditional classroom. Bear in mind that public education has only been around for about a hundred years in our country. In evolutionary terms that is a very short period of time. In essence, children were suddenly required to sit still for long periods of time after having evolved for thousands of years with no such requirement being enforced on such a regular basis.

It is a wonder that so many children get by as well as they do in school, considering that they risk accumulating enough sir to be tarred with the ADHD label if they "...are easily distracted by irrelevant stimuli and frequently interrupt ongoing tasks to attend to trivial noises or events that are usually and easily ignored by others..." So, a child who is more interested in anything else, or becomes involved in anything other than, what his teachers want them to do, can be regarded as meeting part of the ADHD criteria. In evolutionary terms, humans were rewarded by surviving when they were alert to their environment, when they picked up on stimuli that might represent a threat. The alert ones stood a better chance of surviving, while the ones with compliant, placid temperaments—as educators like to see rooms filled with—stood a better chance of getting eaten.

Lest you think school, home, and work settings are the only ones where ADHD signs are picked up, be aware that, "In social settings, inattention may be expressed as frequent shifts in conversation, not listening to others, not keeping one's mind on conversations, and not following details of rules of games or activities." Who knew that parties could be an ADHD minefield? Who would ever have thought in the past that evidence of disorder could be found in how children play with each other?

As easy as it is to diagnose problems with attention, activity levels are even more prone to abuse.

> *Hyperactivity may be manifested by fidgetiness or squirming in one's seat (Criterion A2a), by not remaining seated when expected to do so (Criterion A2b), by excessive running or climbing in situations where it is inappropriate (Criterion A2c), by having difficulty playing or engaging quietly in leisure activities (Criterion A2d), by appearing to be often 'on the go' or as if 'driven by a motor' (Criterion A2e), or by talking excessively (Criterion A2f).*

Here it becomes especially clear just how easily the basis for a diagnosis can be made that applies to almost any child you want it to, especially in school settings. Here also we see a complete lack of understanding of, or any interest in, how real children function. Particularly offensive is the inference that children are okay, or not okay, depending on how "easy" they are to have around. In effect, children can only safely avoid meeting this criteria and being considered to suffer from a neurological abnormality only by acting like sedentary and placid adults.

How much fidgeting does it take to become a problem? Constant fidgeting, once or twice a day, constantly? And what is a fidget? Can a small amount of movement be considered one, or does it take a lot? As Tony Soprano once asked, "What constitutes a fidget?" Same problem with squirming. If I am doing the evaluating, what is a squirm and how many does it take? Does a slight squirm count, or is there a minimal movement quota? As for not remaining seated when one is supposed to, maybe the problem is with adults who place unreasonable expectations on active kids. And God forbid a child should climb when it is forbidden, no matter how alluring the object being ascended is. When does this running or climbing become excessive? The obvious answer is—whenever an adult is disturbed by it. Anybody who expects kids to play or engage in leisure activities quietly is simply not being rational. Sure, some kids do, but other children make more noise. Remember, half of all children will climb, fidget, squirm, and run more than "normal" (the average), some will do so a lot more. Criterion A2f adds, "talking excessively" to the mix. When does talking become excessive? Is it really more the timing of the talking and what the kids say that counts? Is it the content of their speech that does it, the volume? Again, with no clear guide as to quantity or intensity, it comes down to the subjective opinions and intentions of whoever is doing the evaluating.

The criteria for impulsivity is no improvement, "Impulsivity manifests itself as impatience, difficulty in delaying responses, blurting out answers before questions have been completed (Criterion A2G), and frequently interrupting or intruding on others to the point of causing difficulties in social, academic, or occupational settings (Criterion A2i)." Additional sins include clowning, touching things, and grabbing.

The most striking thing about the DSM IV diagnostic criteria, second only to its complete lack of anything resembling science, is how dependent it is on how children function in school, which is why there is no surprise that the bulk of initial identifications of ADHD candidates come from schools. Maybe we should outfit schools with devices like the "cone of silence" seen in the 60's spy spoof, *Get Smart*. A sound-proof cylinder could be lowered over the desk of any disruptive, distracting child.

Impulsivity is another natural feature of childhood, and it is something children learn to moderate, to differing degrees, as they get older. This is a normal part of development, and impulsive behaviors are normal, too, occuring with more or less frequency in different children. The human brain does not stop developing early in childhood, as many used to assume. In fact, significant development occurs in adolescence and one of the things that develops is the capacity for self-regulation.

Thought the initial ADHD diagnosis is primarily driven by the schools and the "undesirable" behaviors of children that they want to contain, the DSM IV says "some" impairment must occur in two or more settings, which means a child can be labeled if he inconveniences adults in more than one place. Yet, the level does not have to be the same, which is a great "out" for educators trying to affix the diagnosis to children. After all, children tend to act like children in more than one setting, so the nasty behaviors seen in one spot will naturally be seen elsewhere, even if not as severe. Read on for more of what the DSM IV has to say:

> It is very unusual for an individual to display the same level of dysfunction in all settings or within the same setting at all times. Symptoms typically worsen in situations that require sustained attention or mental effort or that lack intrinsic appeal or novelty (e.g., listening to classroom teachers, doing class assignment, listening to or reading lengthy materials, or working on monotonous, repetitive tasks). Signs of the disorder may be minimal or absent when the person is receiving frequent rewards for appropriate behavior, is under close supervision, is in a novel setting, is engaged in especially interesting activities,

or is in a one-to-one situation (e.g., the clinicians office). The symptoms are more likely to occur in group situations (e.g., in playgroups, classrooms, or work environments). The clinician should therefore gather information from multiple sources (e.g., parents, teachers) and inquire about the individual's behavior in a variety of situations within each setting (e.g., doing homework, having meals).

So, even though the symptoms should occur in at least two settings, they can be more severe in one of them. What this translates into is that the child who is considered a headache in his school can easily be found to display the same symptoms at home. Sure, the symptoms are worse in school because, as stated above, the expectations bring out the underlying disorder. At home, where more freedom is allowed, the symptoms are naturally less pronounced, but still can be seen. Of course they can; they can be found in just about any child. In addition, if the specific criteria is being hunted for, evidence of it is sure to be found. Kids do act like kids in more than one location. Even the best parents, then, who are informed by the schools that their child might be ADHD, can be talked into thinking the offenses exist in more than just the school, especially if the child has the kind of temperament that makes them likely to be included in the catch-all ADHD net.

As far as the symptoms worsening in situations that require sustained attention or mental effort, the DSM goes on to say that signs of the disorder may go away if the person is "receiving frequent rewards for appropriate behavior..." It is not the ability to pay attention that matters, then, it is paying attention to what you are supposed to, whether or not the subject holds any interest for you.

No account at all is made for the differing interests of children or the fact that what they often are called on to give attention to in school really is boring. Using the ADHD criteria, a school can be as dull as it wants to be, for a mechanism exists for tagging the child with the problem, even though the real problem is a lack of educational initiative and effort.

Signs of ADHD are absent in all of us when we are doing things that are rewarding. Naturally, though, there is no mention of a child's need for interesting environments influencing how he acts in a dull one. The preference is to drug the ones whose actions point out our own shortcomings. And why not? Children are the ones in the equation with the least power. Within the ADHD diagnostic criteria we see a complete lack of respect or concern for children as unique individuals with a wide range of temperaments, abilities, and interests, none of which are evidence of an organic abnormality or disease.

Take a look back at the reprint of the diagnostic criteria as you consider the three subtypes of ADHD listed below. For the first, a child merely has to display 6 or more of 9 symptoms from two lists. The following two subtypes are even easier because each is confined to only one list. Though symptoms are supposed to be indications of a disorder, all of these can also indicate the actions of a normal kid.

Attention Deficit Hyperactivity Disorder, Combined Type. This diagnosis means that the child exhibits at least 6 of 9 symptoms of inattention plus 6 or more of hyperactivity-impulsivity. The majority of kids who are diagnosed ADHD are labeled this type.

Attention Deficit Hyperactivity Disorder, Predominately Inattentive Type. For this it is only necessary to display 6 or more symptoms of inattention, though there still can be some (less than 6) symptoms of hyperactivity-impulsivity.

Attention Deficit Hyperactivity Disorder, Predominately Hyperactive-Impulsive Type. Six or more symptoms of hyperactivity-impulsivity. Some (less than six) symptoms of inattention may be present.

Notice in the A list that the word "often" is used for every Chinese-menu item listed, with no clarification as to what "often" means. Go through this list yourself. I bet most readers could easily give themselves a diagnosis of ADHD if they wanted to, just as more and more adults are. The criteria are so broad and subjective that any child who is troublesome can be labeled as ADHD, with the goal of medicating them to eliminate, or at least make tolerable, the troublesome behaviors. Bear in mind that a child whose natural temperament makes them a poor fit for school, and who shows it through their actions, will behave in exactly the ways listed in the criteria.

Now, a child who does not fall into the three subtypes listed above is not off the ADHD hook, though it seems that at least one of them could be applied to anybody, with a little creativity, who is breathing. For these children we have Attention Deficit Hyperactivity Disorder Not Otherwise Specified. This allows us to label people whose age of onset was later than 7 and, "Individuals with clinically significant impairment who present with inattention and whose symptom pattern does not meet the full criteria for the disorder but have a behavioral pattern marked by sluggishness, daydreaming, and hypoactivity." Here the DSM IV achieves a level of absurdity that would be comic if the ramifications for children were not so serious. This category enables clinicians to diagnosis ADHD in children who *are not active enough* and happen to pay insufficient attention, but not so insufficient as to warrant the inattentive subtype.

This makes it possible to assume a child who is bored, but sits quietly instead of acting out, is suffering from a brain malfunction. What it comes down to is that any child in school who is not exactly as attentive as educators want her to be, whether she acts out or not, or even shows difficulty in paying attention or not, can be referred for a diagnosis. The child who simply decides not to be engaged "appropriately" can be attacked with drugs. Does that sound too harsh? Read this, under the "recording procedures" section for ADHD, "When an individual's symptoms do not currently meet full criteria for the disorder and it is unclear whether criteria for the disorder have previously been met, Attention-Deficit/Hyperactivity Disorder Not Otherwise Specified should be diagnosed." The ADHD criteria have been made broad enough so that any troublesome child can qualify.

The DSM IV's diagnostic criteria for ADHD were developed by a committee put together by the American Psychiatric Association, who also publish the DSM. It consisted of 12 psychiatrists, 4 psychologists, and no pediatricians, which means that nobody with ongoing experience of primary care issues in children participated. Despite this glaring lack of input, the Task Force of the American Academy of Pediatrics accepted the DSM IV as the basis for making ADHD determinations in children. But, easy as those criteria are to use as the basis for diagnosing almost anybody, a 1999 report by Wasserman and associates [3] "Identification of Attentional and Hyperactivity Problems in Primary Care" which surveyed 401 primary care pediatricians, revealed that only 38.3% used the DSM IV in making ADHD determinations. What does this mean? Probably that even the minimal requirements of the DSM are not met in practice and that children are being diagnosed as ADHD for just about anything that annoys adults, be it trouble finishing homework, not controlling their impulses well enough, the refusal to follow directions, moving around too much, not playing nicely with other children, talking back, and so on. In the real world, there don't have to be 6 of 9 symptoms noted, nor do these have to occur in two settings. All that is necessary is that a child becomes difficult in any way, major or minor—particularly in school.

The diagnostic criteria from the DSM are followed in developing materials used by educators to identify and evaluate their students for ADHD, then used to convince parents that their children need to be seen by their physicians for an assessment of ADHD. Of course, schools are very interested in, often insistent on, providing their input to physicians they hope will rely on it to make the diagnosis and write the prescription. All too many do and, if one physician doesn't, many schools will help parents find another who will.

As we see over and over in the true stories from parents featured throughout this book, once a child has been identified as ADHD a school can be relentless in following though until the pills start going down the targeted child's throat, no matter if parents are in agreement or not. Should a parent resist they are likely to be regarded as foolish, undereducated incompetents whose blind stupidity threatens their child's future. Seeing themselves as enlightened and possessed of special knowledge and insight the resistant parent is not privy to, educators will resort to punishing or ostracizing the child in order to pressure the parent, and manipulate, misinform, threaten, and bully parents in the name of accomplishing what they think is right. The DSM criteria are so easy to use and abuse that unethical teachers, school psychologists, counselors, social workers, and various other professionals become tyrants, drunk with the power to abuse any troublesome child, or entire family, at will.

In *The Magic Feather*, [4] a book about special education, authors Lori and Bill Granger sum up a common attitude toward parents by quoting Lawrence Lieberman, a special educator at Boston College, from an article that originally appeared in the *Journal of Learning Disabilities* in January of 1983. Though his formula for bullying parents addresses getting parents to accept special education services it is the same approach used to force the ADHD diagnosis, often part of the special education package:

A problem has arisen that had not been obvious or even in evidence prior to the proliferation of special education services. It has the potential to be one of the greatest sources of frustration to special educators. It is the unwillingness of some parents to allow services to be provided regardless of perceived need and availability of these services...Too many educators are willing to take no for an answer, without exploring the possibilities inherent in more aggressive behavior. How many phone calls are made? How many school meetings are called? How many different teachers and administrators continuously present the same viewpoint (that the child needs help)? Finally, how much pressure is exerted on the parents? There have been cases where school systems have asked for a hearing because the parents are unwilling to sign an educational plan. It is obvious there are times when educators must assert themselves and preserve their own rights as professionals to pursue their profession.

Over the years we have heard from countless parents all over the country who have been victims of the abusive practices outlined above, relentlessly hounded to label and medicate their children, scorned and punished when they do not, and the practice continues. Schools use the absurd DSM criteria to peg a child as abnormal, which provides them what they believe to be a legitimate excuse for berating parents until their child's body is invaded by toxins that make him more compliant.

For those teachers, psychologists, counselors, and administrators of today bent on labeling children as ADHD, the service they want comes in the form of pills that damp down whatever student behaviors are troubling to them, and too many view their right to pursue their profession as the right to badger uncooperative parents into drugging their child in order to make the conduct of their profession in the classroom easier. Never mind that there is no evidence the educational profession is doing a particularly good job to begin with. As the National Commission on Excellence in Education stated in 1983, in words that ring with even more truth today, "If an unfriendly foreign power had attempted to impose on America the mediocre educational performance that exists today, we might well have viewed it as an act of war."

A quote from Carl Jung at the beginning of *The Magic Feather* is a wonderful message for diagnosis and drug happy educators and physicians, "If there is anything that we wish to change in the child, we should first examine it and see whether it is not something that could be better changed in ourselves."

Teachers supplying physicians with the ammunition for an ADHD diagnosis is not a one-way street. Included in a set of recommendations for physicians that comes from the American Medical Association [5] are the following, "The AMA encourages physicians and medical groups to work with schools to improve teachers' abilities to recognize ADHD and appropriately recommend that parents seek medical evaluation..." and "The AMA reaffirms Policy 100.975, to work with the FDA and the DEA to help ensure that appropriate amounts of methylphenidate and other schedule II drugs are available for clinically warranted patent use."

Both recommendations are reprehensible. The first further encourages teachers, who are already much too enthusiastic about practicing medicine without a license, to assist in making a fraudulent diagnosis that leads to the prescription of drugs in the same category as cocaine and speed, exactly what schools tell children *not* to take. The second pushes these addictive drugs on a population of children free of any demonstrable physical abnormality.

Another abusive ploy that comes from the schools and is often accompanied by the participation of physicians who should know better is to suggest a drug trail when parents resist the DSM criteria educators have identified in their children. In another example of practicing medicine without a license, parents are urged to try out some ADHD medication. If it works, then the kid had ADHD all along and it has now been confirmed. If not, well, at least now we know for sure. Sound reasonable? It isn't. Because stimulants affect almost everybody the same way, a response to them can be counted on. All that proves is that stimulants affect our brains and behaviors, not that a student has the mythical ADHD.

Using the behaviors seen in the DSM as an excuse to drug children into submission is nothing new. In the 19th century mothers with difficult babies could give them a "soothing syrup" containing laudanum, which is a mixture of alcohol and opium, and the baby would quiet right down. Some babies became addicted, others were soothed to death. The Pure Food and Drug Act of 1905 was supposed to stop this kind of chemical abuse, but now we see the practice is back today, officially sanctioned and promoted and putting far more children at risk that soothing syrups ever did.

A 19th century mother fond of soothing syrup would see today's DSM criteria as being chock full of the very excuses she used, i.e., a child acting impulsively, not paying attention like he should, or just plain being on the go all the time. In both cases, childhood itself is viewed as a disease. In an excellent editorial on this phenomenon, John Silber, Chancellor of Boston University, said in the April 12, 2001 edition of the *Boston Herald*, "Until fairly recently, it was recognized that the transition between babyhood and adulthood was not entirely smooth. Children, in fact, acted up. And their parents had as their duty to explain to them why adults cannot act up."

When schools use unscientific criteria to get children diagnosed and drugged, they cheat children out of the opportunity to draw on the resources they possess to change, adapt, and cope with their environments. Instead of recognizing the difficulties that come along with the maturation process and helping students navigate a healthy course, educators label this normal process as a disease when it conflicts with what they want out of the students. Instead of building a child's confidence in her ability to grow into a successful adult, they undermine it by insisting a neurological abnormality exists whenever the child annoys them, teaching the child they need a pill to function like a normal person. As Silber goes on to say, "...more and more children are being given chemically derived personalities and insulated from stresses and perceptions that are part of maturation." This is a complete perversion of the educational mission, one that is built on a perversion of science.

The DSM criteria also offer parents an easy way out. Ritalin, Adderall, etc. do result in behavioral changes that make most children who take them more manageable in the short run. Because parents are routinely misinformed about ADHD (told it is a chemical imbalance or neurological disorder when nothing of the sort has ever been shown) and the true risks of the medications that follow the label, the cost/benefit comparison that goes into making the decision is distorted. And, medicating requires less time and effort that addressing a child's real needs. In the conclusion of Silber's editorial he tells us, "The skyrocketing increase in the prescription of Ritalin and its competitors to children as young as 2 suggests the dreadful possibility that more and more parents are preferring to dope their children rather than to deal with them. This nightmare prospect grows not out of poverty but unprecedented wealth. It is the most recent illustration of Juvenal's maxim that "luxury is more ruthless than war.""

One of the statements from the National Institutes of Health after their Consensus Development Conference of 1998 was that "a more consistent set of diagnostic procedures and practice guidelines is of utmost importance." To date, that has not happened. The one panel member who was a primary care pediatrician said, "The diagnosis is a mess." Despite these facts, the "mess" that is the DSM IV diagnostic criteria continues to be a powerful mechanism for getting children identified and evaluated for ADHD, with the result that millions are getting medicated whether the prescribing physicians follow the criteria or not.

In 1992 Kirk and Kutchins [6] made some excellent points that can be applied to the DSM as a whole, not just the ADHD diagnosis, "The language used to present these criteria and procedures exudes the spirit of technical rationality. The diagnosis comes with its unique code number; references to unspecified research about 'discriminating power' and national field trials; and defined levels of severity. Through these criteria, describing common, everyday behaviors of children, the rhetoric of science transforms them into what are purported to be objective symptoms of mental disorder. On closer inspection, however, there is nothing that is objective about the diagnostic criteria."

The DSM's diagnostic criteria for ADHD look like the creation of somebody who observed a group of normal children in school and tried to figure out a mechanism for making a disease out of the more irritating, yet normal, behaviors children exhibit, with an eye toward creating as many patients as possible. Testifying at the NIH Consensus Conference Dr. William Carey,

a top pediatric researcher and writer on the subject of temperament in children, said, "...What is now most often described
as ADHD in the United States appears to be a set of normal
behavior variations...This discrepancy leaves the validity of the
construct in doubt."

As invalid as the construct is, children diagnosed with ADHD
are assumed to often have other problems, too. Features said to
be associated with ADHD include "...low frustration tolerance,
temper outbursts, bossiness, stubbornness, excessive and frequent
insistence that requests be met, mood lability, demoralization,
dysphoria, rejection by peers, and poor self-esteem. Academic
achievement is often markedly impaired and devalued, typically
leading to conflict with the family and with school authorities."
The DSM IV tells us that approximately half of all children with
ADHD also have Oppositional Defiant Disorder or Conduct
Disorder. This is no surprise when you see the diagnostic criteria
for them (provided below) and realize that they are additional
excuses for labeling kids who resist adult authority. God forbid
there should be any good reason for them acting this way.

Notice that, although some of the criteria do represent serious problems, as with using weapons, physical cruelty, forcing
another into sexual activity, and property destruction, the criteria
are also wide open and can be used to label children who should
not be considered disordered at all. Needing only a minimum of
three criteria, a child could be diagnosed for Conduct Disorder
without doing anything too horrible.

If one is not quite up to the standards of Conduct Disorder,
there is always Oppositional Defiant Disorder, which is ideal for
teenagers who resist adult authority and do not want to conform
to prevailing norms. In fact, as you look through that one, think
back on if you could have been labeled that when younger. In
many ways it serves as a definition of adolescent behavior that
could be called "Normal teenage ways of acting that we adults
did ourselves but now find very aggravating." The diagnostician is
directed to consider a criterion only if it occurs more than is typi-

cal. If typical means the average, does that mean the 50% of kids above that point meet the criteria?

Look again and replace "adults" with children in criteria (2) and (3) and you will find that we now have a suitable diagnosis for children to apply to many of us annoying adults.

Finally, if Conduct Disorder or Oppositional Defiant Disorder cannot be achieved, even if we stretch things a bit, we can always resort to Disruptive Behavior Disorder Not Otherwise Specified:

> *This category is for disorders characterized by conduct or oppositional defiant behaviors that do not meet the criteria for Conduct Disorder or Oppositional Defiant Disorder. For example, include clinical presentations that do not meet full criteria either for Oppositional Defiant Disorder or Conduct Disorder, but in which there is clinically significant impairment.*

Once again it seems clear that any child who is a disturbance to adults can be labeled as mentally ill, with no consideration that part of what might be happening is a rebellion against people foolish enough to use demeaning labels so recklessly.

Diagnostic criteria for Conduct Disorder

A. A repetitive and persistent pattern of behavior in which the basic rights of others or major age-appropriate societal norms or rules are violated, as manifested by the presence of three (or more) of the following criteria in the past 12 months, with at least one criterion present in the last 6 months:

<u>Aggression to people and animals</u>

(1) often bullies, threatens, or intimidates others

(2) often initiates physical fights

(3) has used a weapon that can cause serious physical harm to others (e.g., a bat, brick, broken bottle, knife, gun)

(4) has been physically cruel to people

(5) has been physically cruel to animals

(6) has stolen while confronting a victim (e.g., mugging, purse snatching, extortion, armed robbery)

(7) has forced someone into sexual activity

Destruction of property

(8) has deliberately engaged in fire setting with the intention of causing serious damage

(9) has deliberately destroyed others' property (other than by fire setting)

Deceitfulness or theft

(10) has broken into someone else's house, building, or car

(11) often lies to obtain goods or favors or to avoid obliga tions (i.e., "cons" others)

(12) has stolen items of nontrivial value without confronting a victim (e.g., shoplifting, but without breaking and enter ing; forgery)

Serious Violations of Rules

(13) often stays out at night despite parental prohibitions, be ginning before age 13 years

(14) has run away from home overnight at least twice while living in parental or parental surrogate home (or once without returning for a lengthy period)

(15)   is often truant from school, beginning before age 13 years

B. The disturbance in behavior causes clinically significant impairment in social, academic, or occupational functioning.

C. If the individual is age 18 years or older, criteria are not met for Antisocial Personality Disorder.

Diagnostic criteria for Oppositional Defiant Disorder

A. A pattern of negativistic, hostile, and defiant behavior lasting at least 6 months, during which four (or more) of the following are present:

(1) often loses temper

(2) often argues with adults

(3) often actively defies or refuses to comply with adults' requests or rules

(4) often deliberately annoys people

(5) often blames others for his or her mistakes or misbehavior

(6) is often touchy or easily annoyed by others

(7) is often angry and resentful

(8) is often spiteful or vindictive

> **Note:** *Consider a criterion met only if the behavior occurs more frequently than is typically observed in individuals of comparable age and developmental level.*

B. The disturbance in behavior causes clinically significant impairment in social, academic, or occupational functioning.

C. The behaviors do not occur exclusively during the course of a psychotic or Mood Disorder.

D. Criteria are not met for Conduct Disorder, and, if the individual is age 18 years or older, criteria are not met for Antisocial Personality Disorder.

The above disorders, like ADHD, were voted into existence by committees, but a group of like-minded individuals does not a scientific diagnosis make. The science writer Arthur C. Clarke reminds us that, "Science, unlike politics or diplomacy, does not depend on consensus or expediency—it progresses by openminded probing, rigorous questioning, independent thought and, when the need arises, being bold enough to say that the emperor has no clothes." The public has been deceived by 40 years of references to hyperactivity, minimal brain damage, ADD, ADHD, etc. as neurologic, pathologic, biologically based, or chemical imbalances, and none of it could pass the test of science. Indeed, the emperor is ugly, and it is not a pretty sight.

If ADHD-labeled kids could be considered to have oppositional and conduct disorders, then why not the whole gamut of disorders that used to be diagnosed almost exclusively in adults? And so, with huge investments made by pharmaceutical companies, the collusion of psychiatry and education, and the persistent misinforming of parents, the net has been widened. Now we have millions of children diagnosed with anxiety and bipolar disorders, as being obsessive compulsive and depressed.

The diagnoses are made based on adult criteria in the DSM but, as with ADHD (which at least is geared to kids), the actual diagnoses are usually made much more loosely, after a brief visit to a physician who couldn't possibly have gained a feel for what is going on in a child's life in so short a period of time.

Below is the DSM-IV entry for depression [7] in adults. Notice that it leaves no room for consideration of a child's environment. This is not just because it is an adult diagnosis. The ADHD diagnosis, specific to children, ignores environment also. Why? Because the point here is to create patients, not understand human beings. A good clinician evaluating a child will, of course, take environment into account. But the exploding numbers of

children receiving almost instant diagnoses of depression tells us
that there are not nearly enough good clinicians around.

Diagnosis of Major Depressive Disorder, Single Episode

A. The person experiences a single major depressive episode:

1. For a major depressive episode a person must have experienced at least five of the nine symptoms below for the same
   two weeks or more, for most of the time almost every day,
   and this is a change from his/her prior level of functioning.
   One of the symptoms must be either (a) depressed mood, or
   (b) loss of interest.

   a. Depressed mood. For children and adolescents, this may
      be irritable mood.

   b. A significantly reduced level of interest or pleasure in
      most or all activities.

   c. A considerable loss or gain of weight (e.g., 5% or more
      change of weight in a month when not dieting). This may
      also be an increase or decrease in appetite. For children,
      they may not gain an expected amount of weight.

   d. Difficulty falling or staying asleep (insomnia), or
      sleeping more than usual (hypersomnia).

   e. Behavior that is agitated or slowed down. Others should
      be able to observe this.

   f. Feeling fatigued, or diminished energy.

   g. Thoughts of worthlessness or extreme guilt
      (not about being ill).

   h. Ability to think, concentrate, or make decisions is
      reduced.

     i. Frequent thoughts of death or suicide (with or without a specific plan), or attempt of suicide.

2. The person's symptoms do not indicate a mixed episode.

3. The person's symptoms are a cause of great distress or difficulty in functioning at home, work, or other important areas.

4. The person's symptoms are not caused by substance use (e.g., alcohol, drugs, medication), or a medical disorder.

5. The person's symptoms are not due to normal grief or bereavement over the death of a loved one, they continue for more than two months, or they include great difficulty in functioning, frequent thoughts of worthlessness, thoughts of suicide, symptoms that are psychotic, or behavior that is slowed down (psychomotor retardation).

B. Another disorder does not better explain the major depressive episode.

C. The person has never had a manic, mixed, or a hypomanic episode (unless an episode was due to a medical disorder or use of a substance).

Isn't it amazing that the one nod to childhood in the above criteria comes in having being irritable replace exhibiting a depressed mood? And what does irritable mean? Whatever the beholder of the offending behavior wants it to. Aside from the death of friends or relatives, no mention is made of factors that cause stress, sadness, and feelings of being depressed. Children diagnosed as depressed are usually responding to something disturbing in their environments. To act sad, irritable, feel worthless, even suicidal are normal responses to, say, divorce, family dysfunction, a change that is difficult to adjust to, and many other things. These things are mostly caused by adults and it is adults who must make the changes that lead to improved emotional functioning in the child. Instead, what happens is that yet more difficulties of human life are labeled as diseases, and normal children acting in normal ways are told they are the sick ones who need medication.

If a child does not qualify for major depression but is gloomy much of the time and experiences little joy in his life, there is a milder form of depression to diagnose and drug them for, dysthymic disorder. As you read through the criteria below, again keep in mind all the life events that cause these symptoms in children.

Diagnosis of Dysthymic Disorder

A. A person has depressed mood for most the time almost every day for at least two years. Children and adolescents may have irritable mood, and the time frame is at least one year

B. While depressed, a person experiences at least two of the following symptoms:

   1. Either overeating or lack of appetite

   2. Sleeping to much or having difficulty sleeping

   3. Fatigue, lack of energy

   4. Poor self-esteem

   5. Difficulty with concentration or decision making

   6. Feeling hopeless

C. A person has not been free of the symptoms during the two-year time period (one-year for children and adolescents).

D. During the two-year time period (one-year for children and adolescents) there has not been a major depressive episode.

E. A person has not had a manic, mixed, or hypomanic episode.

F. The symptoms are not present only during the presence of another chronic disorder.

G. A medical condition or the use of substances (i.e., alcohol, drugs, medication, toxins) do not cause the symptoms.

H. The person's symptoms are a cause of great distress or difficulty in functioning at home, work, or other important areas.

Similar to depression but with the added feature of appearing manic (the disorder used to be called manic depressive) is bipolar disorder, which has become a popular diagnosis to make in children recently. In practice this gets applied to any child with variations in mood that are bothersome.

It is interesting to note that in schools children being educated about illegal drugs (as opposed to the legal ones their schools promote with an efficiency an drug dealer would envy) are told that marijuana is a "gateway drug," meaning that if they take it they are likely to move on to something stronger and more dangerous. But it is with psychiatric drugs and diagnoses that we see the gateway effect employed to much greater affect. Once a child is diagnosed and drugged for ADHD they are in grave danger of being labeled with something more severe and forced to consume drugs that are more dangerous and powerful. The more drugs they are given the more truly abnormal they become because these drugs represent the first real disease to attack their bodies and brains.

Here are the DSM's two forms of bipolar disorder [8], which form the basis for the diagnosis of children—with plenty of room left for creative applications.

Diagnosis of Bipolar I Disorder

A. A person experiences a current or recent episode that is manic, hypomanic, mixed, or depressed.

1. To be a manic episode, for at least one week a person's mood must be out of the ordinary and continuously heightened, exaggerated, or irritable.

2. At least three of the following seven symptoms have been significant and enduring. If the mood is only irritable, then four symptoms are required:

    a. Self-esteem is excessive or grandiose.

    b. The need for sleep is greatly reduced.

    c. Talks much more than usual.

    d. Thoughts and ideas are continuous and without a pattern or focus.

    e. Easily distracted by unimportant things.

    f. An increase in purposeful activity or productivity, or behaving and feeling agitated.

    g. Reckless participation in enjoyable activities that create a high risk for negative consequences (e.g., extensive spending sprees, sexual promiscuity).

3. The person's symptoms do not indicate a mixed episode.

4. The person's symptoms are a cause of great distress or difficulty in functioning at home, work, or other important areas. Or, the symptoms require the person to be hospitalized to protect the person from harming himself/herself or others. Or, the symptoms include psychotic features (hallucinations, delusions).

5. The person's symptoms are not caused by substance use (e.g., alcohol, drugs, medication), or a medical disorder.

B. Unless this is a first single manic episode there has been at least one manic, mixed, hypomanic, or depressive episode.

1. For a major depressive episode a person must have experienced at least five of the nine symptoms below for the same two weeks or more, for most of the time almost every day, and this is a change from his/her prior level of functioning. One of the symptoms must be either (a) depressed mood, or (b) loss of interest:

   a. depressed mood. For children and adolescents, this may be irritable mood

   b. a significantly reduced level of interest or pleasure in most or all activities

   c. a considerable loss or gain of weight (e.g., 5% or more change of weight in a month when not dieting). This may also be an increase or decrease in appetite. For children, they may not gain an expected amount of weight

   d. difficulty falling or staying asleep (insomnia), or sleeping more than usual (hypersomnia)

   e. behavior that is agitated or slowed down. Others should be able to observe this

   f. feeling fatigued, or diminished energy

   g. thoughts of worthlessness or extreme guilt (not about being ill)

   h. ability to think, concentrate, or make decisions is reduced.

   i. frequent thoughts of death or suicide (with or without a specific plan), or attempt of suicide.

2. The person's symptoms do not indicate a mixed episode.

3. The person's symptoms are a cause of great distress or difficulty in functioning at home, work, or other important areas.

4. The person's symptoms are not caused by substance use (e.g., alcohol, drugs, medication), or a medical disorder.

5. The person's symptoms are not due to normal grief or bereavement over the death of a loved one, they continue for more than two months, or they include great difficulty in functioning, frequent thoughts of worthlessness, thoughts of suicide, symptoms that are psychotic, or behavior that is slowed down (psychomotor retardation).

C. Another disorder does not better explain the episode.

Diagnosis of Bipolar II Disorder

A. The person currently has, or in the past has had at least one major depressive episode:

1. For a major depressive episode a person must have experienced at least five of the nine symptoms below for the same two weeks or more, for most of the time almost every day, and this is a change from his/her prior level of functioning. One of the symptoms must be either (a) depressed mood, or (b) loss of interest:

    a. depressed mood; for children and adolescents, this may be irritable mood

    b. a significantly reduced level of interest or pleasure in most or all activities

    c. a considerable loss or gain of weight (e.g., 5% or more change of weight in a month when not dieting), this may also be an increase or decrease in appetite; for children, they may not gain an expected amount of weight.

    d. difficulty falling or staying asleep (insomnia), or sleeping more than usual (hypersomnia)

    e. behavior that is agitated or slowed down; others should be able to observe this

f.   feeling fatigued, or diminished energy

g.   thoughts of worthlessness or extreme guilt
(not about being ill)

h.   ability to think, concentrate, or make decisions is
reduced

i.   frequent thoughts of death or suicide (with or without
a specific plan), or attempt of suicide.

2.   The person's symptoms do not indicate a mixed episode.

3.   The person's symptoms are a cause of great distress or difficulty in functioning at home, work, or other important areas.

4.   The person's symptoms are not caused by substance use (e.g.,
alcohol, drugs, medication), or a medical disorder.

5.   The person's symptoms are not due to normal grief or bereavement over the death of a loved one, they continue for
more than two months, or they include great difficulty in
functioning, frequent thoughts of worthlessness, thoughts
of suicide, symptoms that are psychotic, or behavior that is
slowed down (psychomotor retardation).

B.   The person currently has, or in the past has had at least one
hypomanic episode:

1.   for a hypomanic episode a person's mood must be out of
the ordinary and continuously heightened, exaggerated, or
irritable for at least four days

2.   at least three of the following seven symptoms have been
significant and enduring; if the mood is only irritable, then
four symptoms are required:

a. self-esteem is excessive or grandiose

b. the need for sleep is greatly reduced

   c. talks much more than usual

   d. thoughts and ideas are continuous and without a pattern or focus

   e. easily distracted by unimportant things

   f. an increase in purposeful activity or productivity, or behaving and feeling agitated

   g. reckless participation in enjoyable activities that create a high risk for negative consequences (e.g., extensive spending sprees, sexual promiscuity).

3. The episode is a substantial change for the person and uncharacteristic of his or her usual functioning.

4. The changes of functioning and mood can be observed by others.

5. The person's symptoms are NOT severe enough to cause difficulty in functioning at home, work, or other important areas. Also, the symptoms neither require the person to be hospitalized, nor are there any psychotic features.

The person's symptoms are not caused by substance use (e.g., alcohol, drugs, medication), or a medical disorder.
C. The person has never experienced a manic or mixed episode.
D. Another disorder does not better explain the episode.
E. The symptoms are a cause of great distress or difficulty in functioning at home, work, or other important areas.

Anxiety disorders have become another major growth area. Below are the DSM criteria for generalized anxiety disorder [9] and obsessive compulsive disorder. Worry and anxiety are normal parts of life and, as with feelings of depression, occur in children in response to something in their environment, which, of course, continues to be ignored. So, here we have another expansion in the territory over which disease is trumping difficulty, another area where children experiencing very real emotional distress are called mentally ill and their symptoms damped down with medications. As always, the children, with nothing wrong with them to begin with, bear all the risk and suffer all the ill effects, while adult run companies and professions accumulate huge profits by abusing them. And what is next? Will children be considered diseased for sleeping late, for their taste in clothes, music, friends? Don't be surprised. After all, the diagnostic criteria are just a committee away.

Diagnostic criteria for 300.02 Generalized Anxiety Disorder

A. Excessive anxiety and worry (apprehensive expectation), occurring more days than not for at least 6 months, about a number of events or activities (such as work or school performance).

B. The person finds it difficult to control the worry.

C. The anxiety and worry are associated with three (or more) of the following six symptoms (with at least some symptoms present for more days than not for the past 6 months). **Note:** Only one item is required in children:

(1) restlessness or feeling keyed up or on edge

(2) being easily fatigued

(3) difficulty concentrating or mind going blank

(4) irritability

(5) muscle tension

(6) sleep disturbance (difficulty falling or staying asleep, or restless unsatisfying sleep).

D. The focus of the anxiety and worry is not confined to features of an Axis I disorder, e.g., the anxiety or worry is not about having a Panic Attack (as in Panic Disorder), being embarrassed in public (as in Social Phobia), being contaminated (as in Obsessive-Compulsive Disorder), being away from home or close relatives (as in Separation Anxiety Disorder), losing weight (as in Anorexia Nervosa), having multiple physical complaints (as in Somatization Disorder), or having a serious illness (as in Hypochondriasis), and the anxiety and worry do not occur exclusively during Posttraumatic Stress Disorder.

E. The anxiety, worry, or physical symptoms cause clinically significant distress or impairment in social, occupational, or other important areas of functioning.

F. The disturbance is not due to the direct physiological effects of a substance (e.g., a drug of abuse, a medication) or a general medical condition (e.g., hyperthyroidism) and does not occur exclusively during a Mood Disorder, a Psychotic Disorder, or a Pervasive Developmental Disorder.

Diagnostic criteria for 300.3 Obsessive-Compulsive Disorder

A. Either obsessions or compulsions:

Obsessions as defined by (1), (2), (3), and (4):

(1) recurrent and persistent thoughts, impulses, or images that are experienced, at some time during the disturbance, as intrusive and inappropriate and that cause marked anxiety or distress

(2) the thoughts, impulses, or images are not simply excessive worries about real-life problems

(3) the person attempts to ignore or suppress such thoughts, impulses, or images, or to neutralize them with some other thought or action

(4) the person recognizes that the obsessional thoughts, impulses, or images are a product of his or her own mind (not imposed from without as in thought insertion).

Compulsions as defined by (1) and (2):

(1) repetitive behaviors (e.g., hand washing, ordering, checking) or mental acts (e.g., praying, counting, repeating words silently) that the person feels driven to perform in response to an obsession, or according to rules that must be applied rigidly

(2) the behaviors or mental acts are aimed at preventing or reducing distress or preventing some dreaded event or situation; however, these behaviors or mental acts either are not connected in a realistic way with what they are designed to neutralize or prevent or are clearly excessive.

B. At some point during the course of the disorder, the person has recognized that the obsessions or compulsions are excessive or unreasonable. **Note:** This does not apply to children.

C. The obsessions or compulsions cause marked distress, are time consuming (take more than 1 hour a day), or significantly interfere with the person's normal routine, occupational (or academic) functioning, or usual social activities or relationships.

D. If another Axis I disorder is present, the content of the obsessions or compulsions is not restricted to it (e.g., preoccupation with food in the presence of an Eating Disorders; hair pulling in the presence of Trichotillomania; concern with appearance in the presence of Body Dysmorphic Disorder; preoccupation with drugs in the presence of a Substance Use Disorder; preoccupation with having a serious illness in the presence of Hypochondriasis; preoccupation with sexual urges or fantasies in the presence of a Paraphilia; or guilty ruminations in the presence of Major Depressive Disorder).

E. The disturbance is not due to the direct physiological effects of a substance (e.g., a drug of abuse, a medication) or a general medical condition.

Specify if:

With Poor Insight: if, for most of the time during the current episode the person does not recognize that the obsessions and compulsions are excessive or unreason able.

Chapter Six

ATTACK OF THE PAPER PUSHERS

*In recent history a disease has been thought of as an entity
established by an underlying biological lesion...in practice
diseases are things whose treatment costs third-party payers
will reimburse.*

- David Healy, M.D.

W hen it comes to childhood psychiatric disorders and medications, pharmaceutical companies influence and shape public consciousness to a frightening degree. Easily observable behaviors that were once known to be normal, like daydreaming or not finishing an assignment, have been redefined as concrete symptoms of a disease. This incredible shift has not occurred because people are gullible or stupid, but because vast resources have been poured into an effort so overwhelming that alternative, or even just sane, voices are drowned out.

Pharmaceutical companies now spend amounts approaching $3 billion a year promoting their wares to the public. They finance drug trials, buy trusted "experts," contribute heavily to supposed advocacy groups, like CHADD (Children and Adults with Attention Deficit Disorders), NAMI (National Alliance for the Mentally Ill) and NARSAD (National Alliance for Research on Schizophrenia and Depression) and employ more Washington lobbyists than there are members of Congress. Never before in medicine has there been such an onslaught, where the flow of information to consumers, be it through physicians, educators, advocacy groups, or the media, is largely controlled by a party (pharmaceutical companies) with a huge financial interest in influencing decision-making and deeper pockets than almost any other industry. It is an effort designed to create patients from normal individuals and sell them drugs they do not need for "diseases" there is no proof they have. People do not fall for this because they are stupid or gullible; their faith and trust in medical professionals and institutions, who have traditionally been assumed to work in our best interests, are being manipulated in a well-orchestrated campaign that seizes on the public assumption of ethical standards and conduct as a resource to be leveraged into enormous cash flows.

A noteworthy feature of the advertising campaigns for ADHD drugs is that their true purpose is usually revealed in the materials presented. How often have you seen pieces on television, radio, parents magazines, or newspapers where smiling parents gaze upon a child who is now doing "better" in school, completing homework with fewer reminders, no longer a behavior problem for his/her teachers? The attraction is behavior management, not the treatment of a disease.

Despite underlying intentions being made clear in advertising propaganda, it remains vital to convince, or at least provide an excuse for, those involved in the diagnostic process that they, by putting children on the path to correct medication, really are doing battle against a harmful condition. Here is a quote from a publication, entitled *Booklet for the Classroom Teacher* by Dr. Larry Silver, [1] that is a good example of what teachers are deluded with:

> *These medications do not cure ADHD. Instead, they appear to work by correcting for a lack of certain necessary brain chemicals in the nervous system. They make the child "normal" by correcting for a neurochemical imbalance. Parents should be aware that these medications do not "drug" or "alter" the brain of the child.*

ADHD drugs do not correct anything. There is nothing abnormal/diseased to correct. They are toxins that seriously alter normal brain functioning, not improve it, and expose them to an

array of unjustifiable risks. These drugs most certainly do drug
the brain of the child—that is how they work, just like cocaine
and speed. This publication is no longer distributed to schools. It
does not need to be. Nowadays the same sort of lies are taught to
prospective teachers as part of the curriculum while they are in
college and graduate school, and also continue to be received in
the form of seminars, continuing education, and training.

CHADD (Children and Adults with Attention-Deficit/Hy-
peractivity Disorder), the largest and most active ADHD advocacy
group, who has long received significant sums of money from pharmaceutical companies and features many of the same Pharma-pur-
chased experts, produces a web site and a series of free publications
for educators, medical professionals, and parents. For example,
one that can be downloaded is called "Attention Deficit Disorder:
Beyond the Myths" and is published by the U.S. Department of
Education [2], who contracted with a private agency to develop
it. As a "FACT" it claims, "Scientific research tells us ADD is a
biologically-based disorder that includes distractibility, impulsiveness, and sometimes hyperactivity." Legitimate scientific research
has never proven any such thing, yet the above lie is presented to
multitudes of parents and educators as a fact.

Harvey Parker, a psychologist who is a co-founder of
CHADD, once had the following suggestion for making it easier
to get kids to take their medicine, "Give the Ritalin pill before
the kid gets up in the morning. Parents sometimes pop it in their
mouth before the eyes are open." Imagine that, poison your child
with a cocaine cousin before he even has a chance to wake up.
Nice suggestion.

There is plenty of propaganda in equally bad places, too, like
the offices of pediatricians. For example, not long ago, I (co-author
Craig Hovey) brought my daughter in for her annual physical and
saw an array of ADHD pamphlets displayed in the waiting area,
all produced and supplied by pharmaceutical companies. Shire,
the company that produces Adderall, had one pushing their once-
a-day version. Opening it to the first page revealed the statement

that, "Stimulant medications have been used successfully and safely to treat ADHD for more than 30 years." This is a lie. There is no evidence of a single lasting benefit experienced by a child who is forced to take amphetamines, and plenty of evidence that giving speed to children is unnecessary and dangerous. Bear in mind from back in Chapter Two that Adderall was already taken off the market, under a different name, back in the 80s because of the dangers it displayed as a diet drug for adults. And now the latest manufacturer of the same amphetamine cocktail has the nerve to call stimulant treatment for children safe!

Below this statement, the next paragraph begins with, "It is believed that medications like Adderall–XR may help restore a chemical balance in the areas of the brain that control our ability to focus and pay attention to tasks." The notion that ADHD or any other psychiatric diagnosis/condition is the result of a demonstrable chemical imbalance is a lie. What has been proven is that amphetamines "improve" the focus and ability to pay attention for anybody who takes them in the short run, but the risks of the drugs badly outweigh a temporary effect that does not last. Note the language used in the above quote, "It is believed" and "may help." Appearing in a nicely done pamphlet made available in the offices of respected physicians, readers are supposed to think qualified people assessing credible research believe this, but this is simply not the case.

After the manipulative line on how Adderall "works" the next section tells us that, "ADHD is a condition that affects approximately 3 - 7% of school-age children." Condition here is a euphemism for disease, in yet another muddying use of language. But, as we have already seen, ADHD has never been proven to be a disease at all. The drug pushers seek to give the impression that ADHD meets the criteria of a disease, and therefore qualifies for diagnosis and drugs, while, at the same time, using words like "condition" to avoid alarming parents with the notion that their children are sick.

In the same office another pamphlet by the same company, Shire, has a section where they continue their efforts to broaden the patient population to any extreme possible. Traditionally boys, more physically active than girls, have been the primary targets, but more girls are now being tarred and poisoned. How? Shire emphasizes the "inattentive" side of ADHD with girls, telling us these girls "...are the daydreamers whose minds drift in school. They have trouble concentrating and are forgetful and disorganized." Couldn't it just be that their daydreams are more interesting than school? Can't children, who are still developing, after all, be forgiven for being forgetful and disorganized, and maybe helped along in the maturation process, instead of being force-fed amphetamines?

In the above, we again see the pervasive emphasis on school functioning (with no evidence of long-term enhancement of educational outcome) as was repeated in other pamphlets by other pharmaceutical companies for other drugs in the same waiting room. A new twist has been the effectiveness in ADHD drugs "helping" children through structured after-school activities also, which just extends the time children need to act like their placid adult taskmasters instead of being the kids they are. A pamphlet for Concerta tells us that, "ADHD doesn't end when a child's school day does," and gives us examples with parent testimonials. Concerta is a long acting form of methylphenidate (Ritalin), that old standby we already know for a chemical cousin of cocaine. Could you imagine the outrage if cocaine and speed were advertised in doctor offices? Yet, were this to happen, the ethics would be no less shabby than what we see now. In fact, it might be an improvement, as at least parents would be given a better idea of what these drugs really are.

In the pamphlet we learn that Concerta rescued one little boy after his "...symptoms were preventing him from concentrating on the work his first-grade teacher gave him in school and on what his parents were trying to teach him at home." Is Concerta really being presented as a legitimate medication here? No, it is being sold as a performance enhancer with barely a veneer of legitimacy. Later in this same dismal publication we hear of a little girl who was diagnosed with ADHD in kindergarten. "Everything used to be a struggle," her mother is quoted as saying. Further details are revealed with, "Just sitting down was difficult...Any distraction would take her off-task. Sometimes she would forget her afternoon dose of ADHD medicine, and then she would have a hard time focusing and not do her homework." Though not stated in any of these cases, it is not hard to imagine the schools being the ones who initially pushed the ADHD diagnosis. Indeed, the effectiveness of American public schools in the drug pushing business is one of their few success stories.

Lilly, the makers of Strattera (a newer ADHD drug, being aggressively marketed), uses a similar approach in attempting to expand the numbers of adults said to have ADHD. In the April 8, 2004, issue of Parade magazine they had an insert that protruded above the top of a page with this question: "Modern Life or Adult ADHD?" On the page below were a series of one-word questions overlaying a series of pictures of a woman in increasing distress: "Distracted?" and "Disorganized?" and "Frustrated?" Below was the instruction to "Take the Attached Test and Talk with your Doctor." This "test" is a series of six subjective questions and tells you that the right kind of answers to four or more means "...that your symptoms may be consistent with ADHD." In other words, you might behave in ways that parallel an imaginary disease. And what do the questions concern? The usual stuff, like fidgeting, squirming, difficulty getting things in order, wrapping up details, and procrastinating. And how are you supposed to tell the difference between a disease and modern life? By simply deciding you experience these things more often than you want to. But won't your physician shoot this down if you bring in your list of symptoms? A physician who remains true to his/her scientific training will, but more likely they will give you the diagnosis you came for, and maybe even provide you a free sample - one of those starter kits pharmaceutical companies are so generous with.

As ridiculous as the advertisement considered above is, there are innumerable ratings scales and evaluation forms that have been manufactured for use by educators and other professionals that are no better. And these are the kinds of instruments schools employ for their initial ADHD evaluations and use to prod and manipulate parents into bringing their children to pediatricians, family doctors, or child psychiatrists. Because the school-based materials are driven by the same criteria physicians are apt to use, they become short-cuts that allow determinations to be made quickly, usually within the short time periods (15 minutes is common) allowed by health insurance companies. In case after case we've had parents report to us that just relaying subjective conclusions that were delivered to them by a teacher verbally can be enough to garner an ADHD diagnosis when passed on to a physician.

With the popular ADHD evaluation instruments a lasting determination that a child has a neurobiological disorder can be made in minutes, by people with no medical training who can easily wield the deadly forms to label any child they want. How? The stunning fact is that these results are taken seriously.

THE DEVIL IN BLACK AND WHITE

Below is one of the most frequently used and, therefore abused instruments, the Pittsburgh Modified Conners Teacher Rating Scale. [3] The complete form can easily be filled out in minutes. The items necessary to justify a diagnosis of ADHD in a child can be polished off in 20 seconds. And the criteria are even more subjective than those of the DSM IV it is based on. By the time teachers fill these things out, they probably have already made up their minds about the child. Further, if they have a child on their hands they want to "contain," the standards seen here are so loose as to be wide open for manipulation.

Parent after parent share with us their suspicions that the decision had been made before any ratings or evaluations were done, with educators knowing exactly what to do to support their desire for the ADHD label and, more importantly, getting a normal child drugged so they will be easier to manage in class.

PITTSBURGH MODIFIED CONNERS TEACHER RATING SCALE

INSTRUCTIONS: Listed below are items concerning children's behavior or the problems they sometimes have. Read each item carefully and decide how much you think the items describe this child at this time.

Not at All. Just a Little. Pretty Much. Very Much.

1. Fidgeting
2. Hums and makes other odd noises
3. Excitable, impulsive
4. Inattentive, easily distracted
5. Fails to finish things he or she starts
   (Short attention span)
6. Quarrelsome
7. Acts "smart"
8. Temper outburst- behavior explosive and unpredictable
9. Defiant
10. Uncooperative
11. Restless and overactive
12. Disturbs other children
13. Demands must be met immediately – easily frustrated
14. Cries often and easily
15. Mood changes quickly and drastically
16. Fights, hits, punches, etc.
17. Is disliked by other children

18. Frequently interrupts other children's activities

19. Bossy: always telling other children what to do

20. Teases or calls other children names

21. Refuses to participate in group activities

22. Is actively rejected by other children

23. Is simply ignored by other children

24. To what extent is this child's behavior towards peers like that of a normal child?

Very much like a normal child 0 1 2 3 4 5 6 Not at all like a normal child

25. To what extent is this child's behavior towards adults like that of a normal child?

Very much like a normal child 0 1 2 3 4 5 6 Not at all like a normal child

26. To what extent do you find interacting with this child a pleasant experience?

Very pleasant 0 1 2 3 4 5 6 Very unpleasant

Overall, how serious a problem do you think this child has at this time?

NONE   MILD   MODERATE   SEVERE
|____| |____| |_____| |_____|

Please feel free to include any additional comments on the reverse side of this form.

Not every item on the above rating scale deals specifically with ADHD, so let's define the ones that do and go into how they are scored. This scale is a composite of items from two other scales and yields two different sets of answers that are used to generate scores that are then used as the basis for "further assessment," which generally translates into pushing parents into getting their child to a physician who will use the results to make a diagnosis and write a prescription. As we saw in the story of Joy and Paul in the second chapter, educators who do an initial evaluation frequently recommend physicians they know are "friendly" to ADHD. The whole process could be made a lot more efficient, and yield a similar result, if we just gave teachers prescription pads to keep in their desks.

Items that are checked "Not at All" receive a score of "0," a "Just a Little" gets a "1," "Pretty Much" earns a "2," and "Very Much" gives us the highest score, a "3."

The scores from two different sets of questions can be added up to determine whether a child gets referred for "further assessment," meaning they are pushed a step closer to having stimulant drugs pushed on them. The first set, which is the one used for ADHD, consists of items 1–5, with scores of 8 or above justifying that further assessment recommendation, as seen in the actual language, "For screening purposes in classroom settings, a total score of 8...would indicate referral for further assessment..."

Let's see just how horrible a child needs to act in order to enter ADHD territory using this scale. Item #1 is "Fidgeting." As with DSM IV, what constitutes a "fidget" is not defined, which means a teacher can score any child who moves any way they want to. But even if they are a bit more objective, an awful lot of kids will get the higher scores. Why? 50% of children will fidget less and 50% of children will fidget more than average. The categories "Not at All" and "Just a Little" are where the 50% who fidget less will fall. "Pretty Much" and "Very Much" are wide open for that other 50%. The resulting scores of 1 or 2 move the child along the way to an ADHD label, yet children are being scored for acting like normal children who just happen to move around more than average, or whatever the rater decides is normal, which can easily be below the average if the rater wants to stigmatize the child being rated.

#2, "Hums and makes other odd noises" seems too ridiculous to even consider, but we should since our children are judged based on it. It is important to note that a question this silly can be enough to put the score "over the top" in terms of pushing a child down the road to forced drugging. So, if your child happens to like music, or any kinds of sounds at all for that matter, warn them not to repeat them anywhere a label-prone educator might hear. In this question we see the real intention of these scales, to find an excuse that can be used to muzzle innocent, normal children.

#3 is a step closer to sanity only because it is less absurd than #2, "Excitable, Impulsive." Again, 50% of children will be more excitable and impulsive than average. The 50% who are less excitable and impulsive will be scored with zeroes and ones, with any normal child displaying above average quantities of behaviors judged to meet the criteria getting twos and threes. And, again, rating a child on this item depends on the eye of the beholder. A physically inactive teacher who likes placid children could easily mark any child who shows spirit and enthusiasm as "Very Much" in this category. Just how much excitable and impulsive behavior does it take to get twos and threes? Just what is excitable and impulsive behavior anyway? Are there objective measurements we all can share? Are there definite standards? Of course not.

#4 reads, "Inattentive, easily distracted." Starting with the given that 50% of children will be less attentive and more easily distracted than others, at what point do these behaviors put a child in the "Pretty Much" or "Very Much" categories, where a 2 or 3 edge one closer to a ADHD label? Also, isn't it possible that a child could be inattentive or easily distracted because the subject or teacher is boring to them? Maybe something else they are more interested in is occupying their thoughts. For children living through tough times at home, couldn't they be distracted by larger issues that capture their attention instead of what is going on in the classroom? Could the child just have a different learning style than is catered to by a particular teacher? Could they have other learning problems that are being overshadowed by suspicions of ADHD? Or maybe they have a physical problem that interferes with their ability to attend in the classroom? All of the above things are factors that have nothing to do with ADHD, yet any one could be the item that puts a child at, or above, the magic number of 8.

#5 compounds the problem by essentially repeating #4, which means a kid whose lack of attention can be due to any number of factors unrelated to ADHD can be double-counted and cause a child to get exactly that label. It reads, "Fails to finish things he or she starts (short attention span)." Obviously, being inattentive and easily distracted will result in children not finishing what they start and appearing to have a short attention span. Besides, not finishing things and having a short attention span are perfectly normal behaviors for children. The problem is with the educators who will not tolerate normal if it doesn't jibe with how they want kids to act.

With #4 and #5 overlapping, a child given a score of "3" on both is 75% of the way to the ADHD label. In order to hit the magic number 8, all it takes is a "Just a Little" designation on two of the other three items to get the rest of the way there. This means that any child can have a host of things that cause his attention to be insufficient in a teacher's eyes, be it just a difference in temperament, learning style, reaction to a boring setting, or more serious problems like physical impairments or family dysfunction, and be considered ADHD, even though there is nothing neurologically wrong with them.

If this scale, and the many like it, didn't carry so much weight, its outright absurdity would not be such a problem. Clearly it is on so low a diagnostic level as to be on par with practices that predated modern medicine, like bleeding patients to drain them of an evil spirit. What really comes across in the scale is not evidence of any disease, but the degree to which a child's behavior is at odds with the authorities who do not like it. The clash is enough, for whoever carries the lesser weight in the collision loses out, and what weight do children have to throw around?

ADHD is not the only diagnosis made easy with the Conners Scale. Items 6-10 are used to evaluate children for Oppositional Defiant Disorder, with a score of "5" or above being enough to justify further assessment. As with ADHD, there is no notion of there being anything wrong, anywhere, except with the child. A "quarrelsome" kid may in reality have good reasons for arguing, with the quarreling behavior being a healthy and normal response to an unhealthy situation. The "smart" in question 6 must refer to being sarcastic, where the sarcasm is assumed to be a problem residing in the child, with no rational reason for acting that way. Defiant and uncooperative are measuring the same trait so that, just as the ADHD criteria do, a single trait can be enough to justify the label. The Oppositional Defiant label is a means of attacking an uncooperative child under cover of the mental illness assumption, where any kid who doesn't go along with things as they are is assumed to have a disorder.

Next we are going to look at another popular rating scale. This one is likely to be filled out by a school psychologist. Since they are supposed to be more knowledgeable in this area than teachers, there is the reasonable hope that they would be more objective and exercise better judgment. That is not necessarily the case. First of all, they have usually heard the referring teacher's concerns before having anything to do with the child, so their observations are likely to be colored from the outset. Second, they go along with the same DSM IV criteria the simpler teacher scales are based on and, third, the school systems they work for want troublesome kids contained, so they have an incentive here, too, that also may impair their objectivity. Finally, though the instrument below is more involved and less prone to abuse than the Conners Scale, it still is an absurd piece of work that lacks any semblance of scientific credibility.

Below are the questions used in the Attention-Deficit/Hyperactivity Disorder test that is published by PRO-ED. [4] It is widely used and, as with the Conners scale, there are a number of others like it (no surprise, since they are all based on the DSM IV). This scale has subtests for hyperactivity, impulsivity, and inattention, then a section for questions calling for narrative answers and a last section for recommendations and comments. In short, it might be the best of a horrible lot. Here goes.

HYPERACTIVITY SUBTEST

	Not a Problem	Mild Problem	Severe Problem
1. Loud	0	1	2
2. Constantly "on-the-go"	0	1	2
3. Excessive running, jumping, climbing	0	1	2
4. Twisting and wiggling in seat	0	1	2
5. Easily excited	0	1	2
6. Grabs objects	0	1	2
7. Excessive talking	0	1	2
8. Difficulty remaining seated	0	1	2
9. Constantly manipulating objects	0	1	2
10. Inability to play quietly	0	1	2
11. Fidgets	0	1	2
12. Restless	0	1	2
13. Squirms	0	1	2

IMPULSIVITY SUBTEST

	Not a Problem	Mild Problem	Severe Problem

14. Acts before thinking	0	1	2
15. Shifts from one activity to the next	0	1	2
16. Fails to wait for one's turn	0	1	2
17. Difficulty waiting turn	0	1	2
18. Blurts out answers	0	1	2
19. Impulsive	0	1	2
20. Interupts conversations	0	1	2
21. Intrudes on others	0	1	2
22. Does not wait for directions	0	1	2
23. Fails to follow rules of the game	0	1	2

INATTENTION SUBTEST

	Not a Problem	Mild Problem	Severe Problem
24. Poor concentration	0	1	2
25. Fails to finish projects	0	1	2
26. Disorganized	0	1	2
27. Poor planning ability	0	1	2
28. Absentminded	0	1	2
29. Inattentive	0	1	2
30. Difficulty following directions	0	1	2
31. Short attention span	0	1	2

32. Easily distracted	0	1	2
33. Difficulty sustaining attention	0	1	2
34. Difficulty staying on task	0	1	2
35. Difficulty completing tasks	0	1	2
36. Frequently loses things	0	1	2

KEY QUESTIONS

1. Does the person demonstrate six or more symptoms of inattention, or six or more symptoms of hyperactivity, or impulsivity listed in each subtest?

2. Does the person exhibit the behavioral problems in a variety of environments?

3. Does the person demonstrate the behaviors considerably more frequently than do most people of the mental age?

4. Has the person demonstrated the behaviors for at least 6 months?

5. Did the person first demonstrate the behaviors before age 7?

6. Is the person's functioning (at school, home, and work) significantly impaired?

7. Are there other conditions that could possibly be causing the behavioral problems? If yes, what are the conditions?

8. Who has previously evaluated this person and what were the results?

9. What specific interventions have been attempted to treat the person's problems?

10. What additional information needs to be collected?

RECOMMENDATIONS AND COMMENTS

The strength of this rating scale is that the questions and space for recommendations leave a responsible evaluator room to include significant factors, like home environment, that are ignored in stricter adaptations of the DSM IV criteria. The weakness is that it is still based mostly on DSM IV criteria, which leaves it wide open for misuse and is probably what generally happens when it is administered.

Once again, we have an instrument that is completely subjective and allows the evaluator so much leeway that almost any child can be found to be ADHD when that is the goal. Going back to the Hyperactivity Subtest, when does "Loud" become a problem, and where is the dividing line between mild and severe? The same question applies to every item in this section. The answer, I fear, is that the behaviors in question become a problem whenever an adult, usually an educator, decides they are. Once again, the real problem is a lack of tolerance, compassion, understanding, and flexibility on the part of adults.

Though there is serious competition for the most galling item in this section, my vote goes to "Inability to play quietly." At this point, the hostility toward childhood in general becomes apparent. Should we even want children to play quietly? For that matter, is it sane to view squirming, being restless, or fidgeting as problems? Note also the considerable overlap here, so that a physically active child can be rated a severe problem over and over again based on one trait.

Moving on to the Impulsivity Subtest, the most incredible item is "Fails to follow rules of games." Just whose games are these and who decides the rules? Isn't testing rules and learning from breaking them part of normal development? Throughout the ADHD criteria in all its manifestations there is the clear desire to eliminate any behavior that conflicts with adult standards. By doing this, any important source of childhood learning and development is eliminated. Not only are children harmed with a demeaning label and dangerous drugs, but their very evolution as people may be stunted.

The "Fails to follow rules of games" inadvertently gets at what is really going on with the push to label so many children with ADHD. Kids who do not adhere to the rules of their educational environments, a game where the "winners" are rewarded for being quiet, compliant, and doing what they are told with no fuss or bother, are branded as losers whose bad brains interfere with their playing as they should. The intent is to make children play with stacked decks and loaded dice so that the outcomes can be safely predicted by those in charge.

With the Inattention Subtest, once again, the same couple of traits are rated again and again. Again, no consideration is given to why these things may be going on. Particularly obnoxious here, but in all the ratings materials I have seen, is the absence of any consideration that maybe the adults in charge are not doing a good job. To believe only the child could have a problem is the most extreme arrogance. Maybe there is difficulty following directions because the directions are poorly given or often do not make sense. Maybe concentration is poor because the tasks a child is expected to concentrate on don't appear worthy of the effort. Couldn't a child be absent-minded because she is pre-occupied with a more important issue? Isn't it possible for a normal child to be easily distracted when there are alternative stimuli in his environment that interest him more than what his teacher wants him to do?

The "Key Questions" at least give an evaluator the chance to bring in other factors that could account for problems being experienced in school, as seen in question #7. The problem is that these evaluations are rarely done with any other intention than securing a diagnosis for children who exhibit troublesome behaviors. Unfortunately, I doubt there is much concern in practice for other conditions, and the items in the scale prior to the question certainly show no such interest.

The "Recommendations and Comments" section, while it could be an opportunity for thoughtful narrative evaluation, is an opportunity for a subjective evaluator to reinforce the conclusions they probably made before even beginning to fill out the scale.

Though these scales are filled out by non-medical professionals and are supposed to be followed by a medical evaluation in order to make a diagnosis and decision on whether or not to prescribe medication, we have already seen that this procedure is often not followed. Earlier in this book we heard Joy's story of how a teacher had already filled out an evaluation (I do not know if it was an "official" evaluation or one of her own creation), decided that her son had ADHD, and decided on the doctor Joy should take her son to in order to get a prescription. Whatever the evaluation used here, the teacher's mind was already settled on the matter before filling it out, as was the need to have the child medicated, despite the fact that she was completely unqualified to make the determination. This is not unusual. The manipulation of evaluation materials that lack credibility to begin with is common. Considering how many millions of normal children have become victims of the process, it has reached plague-like proportions. The other point to remember is that there are no more reliable testing procedures to be done by a physician. The diagnostic process never improves. With no findings to be had on physical examination, no lab tests, scans, biopsies, x-rays, or any other objective means of discovering or confirming an abnormality, physician assessments are just as subjective as anybody else's and they demean themselves by going along. In medical school physicians-to-be are taught how to make legitimate diagnoses based on real evidence of real disease. Each time any physician makes an ADHD diagnosis they have made a patient of a normal child and have, themselves, failed to make the grade as physicians.

NOT JUST FOR KIDS ANYMORE

ADHD is no longer limited to children. Though formerly thought to be a condition outgrown as children moved through adolescence, with but a few adults continuing to suffer its woes, today's thinking is more along the lines that ADHD is a lifetime affliction. More and more adults are being told, or discovering on their own, that they "have" it. For adults, just like kids, the criterion is so broad that anybody can find herself reflected in it. An extra factor that is very important to building up the adult numbers is that the ADHD diagnosis is an attractive explanation for problems they have been experiencing for years, from relationship difficulties to job instability to the inability to finish a book. We do not deny that these things are problems or represent stressful aspects of life. What we are saying is that none by themselves is evidence of a chemical imbalance, neurological abnormality or disease, that needs to be corrected with stimulants.

"I have ADD, and I love having it," says Dr. Edward Hallowell, who came up with the popular checklist reproduced below for assessing ADHD in adults, the Hallowell Index. [5] Hallowell is the author of *Driven To Distraction* [6] and in it claims, "Once you catch on to what this syndrome is all about, you'll see it everywhere." Dr. Hallowell managed to see it in himself, as did his collaborator for the book, John Ratey. Both are psychiatrists. The criteria below are indeed seen everywhere, not because they indicate any kind of syndrome which, remember, in medicine means the same thing as disease, but because they are common, though often difficult, aspects of the human experience. According to Dr. Hallowell, acting like a normal human being grappling with life's difficulties is evidence of a diagnosable abnormality, an indication that you have a brain disease. As he puts it, "ADD is a neurological syndrome." He also estimated, back in 1994, that 15 million people suffered from it and that two-thirds of children with the affliction continue to be burdened by it as adult. Does he offer any evidence for the above claims? Of course not.

Above the index reads the following note, "Consider a criterion met only if the behavior is considerably more frequent than that of most people of the same mental age."

Does he tell us how to assess what anybody's mental age is? Of course not.

ADD IN ADULTS

1. A sense of underachievement
2. Difficulty getting organized
3. Chronic procrastination or trouble getting started
4. Many projects going simultaneously; trouble with follow-through
5. Tendency to say what comes to mind without necessarily considering the timing or appropriateness of the remark
6. A frequent search for high stimulation
7. An intolerance of boredom
8. Easy distractibility, trouble focusing attention, tendency to tune out or drift away
9. Often creative, intuitive, highly intelligent
10. Trouble in going through established channels, following "proper" procedure
11. Impatient; low tolerance for frustration
12. Impulsive, either verbally or in actions
13. Tendency to worry needlessly, endlessly
14. Sense of impending doom or insecurity
15. Mood swings, mood liability
16. Restlessness
17. Tendency toward addictive behavior

18. Chronic problems with self-esteem

19. Inaccurate self-observation

20. Family history of ADD or other disorders of impulse control or mood

In a note to the enhanced version of the above we are told, "These criteria are based on extensive clinical experience but have not yet been statistically validated by field trials." This means they are solely the author's opinion, an author who believes he himself has a nonexistent disease, that has no scientific basis or validity. If you go through the index and feel enough of the items describe you, which should come as no surprise since we all can see ourselves in them, a feat no more difficult than peering into the bathroom mirror, you are instructed to go to a doctor for further evaluation. How hard do you think it would be to find one who will diagnose you and write a prescription?

THE MARKETING OF MENTAL ILLNESS

Providing the public with information that allowed anybody, young or old, to fit the ADHD mold is a practice that has been copied for a succession of more recently promoted disorders. And why not? ADHD has been a huge moneymaker. To understand how the process works, consider the promotion of the anxiety disorders, social anxiety disorder in particular. Not long ago such a diagnosis was made only when a person suffered from debilitating levels of anxiety, like being so frightened of public places that one barely ever emerged from his apartment. Then, in the mid-90s GlaxoSmithKline, the maker of the antidepressant Paxil, got their drug approved for double duty as an anti-anxiety agent and hired a public relations firm to launch a major promotional campaign. It was hugely successful.

Stories in the media about social anxiety disorder leapt from 50 in 1997-98 to over 1 billion references in just 1999. Almost every story mentioned Paxil as the first and only FDA-approved

162 THE ADHD FRAUD

drug for treatment of it. Very rapidly this little known and rarely diagnosed disorder was being referred to by physicians and in testimonials as the third most common mental illness around. Estimates abounded (with no real evidence) that put the number of sufferers from this one form of anxiety disorder at somewhere over 10 million, a number that included such luminaries as Donny Osmond and professional football player, Ricky Williams, men who were happy to step forward and share their suffering and the wondrous cure for it to be found in a pill.

It was made so easy to get diagnosed for social anxiety disorder that anybody could do it. Now, though Paxil hasn't been shown to provide any lasting benefits and puts whoever takes it at risk for anything from a dry mouth to psychosis, it does give most of those who take it a feeling of increased well-being, at least temporarily. Because this is something people will pay for, diagnostic guidelines are very easy to satisfy. As an example of what is used in practice, look at the following checklist from the Adult Anxiety Clinic of Temple University. [7] The directions say, "If you answer 'yes' to some of these statements, you may benefit from treatment for social anxiety." In other words, if pretty much anything is causing you anxiety, you are ill and need to be medicated. Notice that there are a few items on the checklist that are legitimate reasons for concern. While these appear to give it credibility, the great majority of the social anxiety disordered among us got the label based on the more minor league of the problems.

ANSWER YES OR NO TO EACH OF THE FOLLOWING STATEMENTS:

1) I feel anxious or nervous when making presentations for work or school (or almost always avoid these situations).

2) I feel anxious or nervous when interacting with others (or almost always avoid these situations).

3) I feel anxious or nervous eating or drinking in front of others.

4) I have trouble being assertive with family, friends, or strangers.

5) I have difficulty interacting with authority figures   (i.e., boss or teacher).

6) I have used alcohol or tranquilizers to calm my nerves before interacting with others.

7) I am afraid I will do something to humiliate or embarrass myself in a social situation.

8) I fear being judged as inadequate or incompetent by others.

As is apparent from going through the checklist, it is so open-ended, subjective, and filled with ill-defined terms that most human beings who answered it honestly could easily find a physician to diagnosis them and provide pills to make them feel better, for a little while, until the other shoe drops. Sound familiar? Notice that the above criteria could easily be used to justify drugging a child for anxiety, and it has been, over a million times now.

For an even more blatant example of the marketing of a disorder and its accompanying medication, go to the web site called FeelingBlue.com. On this site there are questionnaires for assessing social anxiety disorder, panic disorder, general anxiety disorder, depression, and obsessive compulsive disorder. Paxil and the other antidepressants are prescribed for all of them. Now, guess whose site this is? GlaxoSmithKline, the company that makes Paxil. Below is their questionnaire for depression. In this case there are 11 questions and they provide you the following directions at the bottom of it, "If you answered 'yes' to 5 or more of these questions, print out this self test and bring it to your doctor." Chances are, your doctor has had the same criteria provided to her, along with plenty of incentives to prescribe Paxil, of course.

As with the anxiety sheets, there are some things on here that genuinely require attention if a person is experiencing them. The incredible rise in the numbers who count themselves among the depressed, however, are primarily driven by the problems that are more normal challenges of everyday life than a threat to it.

ANSWER YES OR NO TO THE FOLLOWING STATEMENTS:

1) Have you been feeling sad, depressed or down most of the time?

2) Have you been less interested and less able to enjoy the things that once gave you pleasure?

3) Have you felt tired or without energy most of the time?

4) Have you had trouble sleeping or do you sleep too much?

5) Have you found it difficult to concentrate or make decisions?

6) Have you had an increase or decrease in appetite or weight?

7) Have you had feelings of worthlessness or guilt?

8) Have you felt frightened or panicky for no apparent reason at all?

9) Have you felt restless and found it difficult to sit still?

10) Have you been feeling anxious or worried?

11) Have you felt like you just cannot go on, or had thought about death or dying?

Pretty easy to go through this list and find five things to check, right? Getting a prescription is often even easier than that, as many physicians do not even bother to follow a list this detailed—and this list is so vague that nearly anybody could be diagnosed as depressed. Bottom line: If you want a diagnosis you will easily find somebody to give it to you, along with prescriptions for drugs. This is the danger of treating subjective lists of behavioral criteria as though they are adequate means of determining the existence of a disease. They are not. A real disease, a real disorder, a real abnormality can be identified objectively. The goal of psychiatric disorders is the opposite, to make the criteria as fuzzy and broad as possible so as to draw from the largest possible pool and create the maximum number of permanent patients.

Is this how we want our children treated?

Chapter Seven

SCIENCE FOR SALE

Drug company gifts and "consulting fees" are so pervasive that in any given field you cannot find an expert who has not been paid off in some way by the industry.

- Nathan Newman, Special Report for
The Nation, **July, 2002**

Pharmaceutical companies who are marketing psychopharmacological treatments have gotten into the business of selling psychiatric illness...The way to sell drugs is to sell psychiatric illness.

- Carl Elliot, University of Minnesota bioethicist

In 1999 the *Boston Globe* revealed that Dr. Martin Keller, head of Brown University's Department of Psychiatry, had received $500,000 the prior year in consulting fees from the very same pharmaceutical companies whose products he praised in medical journals and had used federal funds to study. The striking thing about this story is not that it happened, but how standard the practice has become.

And what of Karen Dineen Wagner, M.D., Ph.D., as a purveyor of science and a patient advocate? Not only is she Professor, and Vice Chair, Department of Psychiatry and Behavioral Sciences, Division of Child and Adolescent Psychiatry, University of Texas Medical Branch, Galveston, she is a consultant to Wyeth-Ayerst, Abbott Laboratories, Bristol-Myers Squibb, Cyberonics, Eli Lilly, Forest Laboratories, GlaxoSmithKline; a member of the speakers bureau of Janssen, Abbott Laboratories, Eli Lilly,

GlaxoSmithKline, Forest Laboratories, Pfizer, and Novartis; a scientific advisory board member for Abbott Laboratories, Eli Lilly, Forest Laboratories, GlaxoSmithKline, Novartis, Otsuka, Janssen, Pfizer, UCB Pharma, and Wyeth-Ayerst, and receives research support from Abbott Laboratories, Bristol-Myers Squibb, Eli Lilly, Forest Laboratories, Novartis, Otsuka, Janssen, Pfizer, UCB Pharma, GlaxoSmithKline, Organon, Pfizer, Wyeth-Ayerst, and the National Institute of Mental Health. [1]

Psychiatry long ago stopped functioning as an independent medical specialty. It is now an arm of the pharmaceutical industry, actively engaged in the effort to make pre-paid results look like science. In *Let Them Eat Prozac*, Dr. David Healy [2] tells us, "Scientific progress in psychiatry has been stalemated because Big Pharma's marketing efforts have overwhelmed the field." If scientific progress has been stalemated, then what is going on? A financial windfall resulting from creating illusions of diseases that pharmaceutical company's products are posited as the answer for. As Dr. Healy told us in his previous book, *The Creation of Psychopharmacology* [3], "The techniques used to market information have developed to the point where significant changes in the mentality of both clinicians and the public can be produced within a matter of a few years."

In regard to children, as we argue throughout this book, the first large-scale attempt at this was with ADHD and the drugs sold to "treat" it. [4]

The success found here has inspired ongoing efforts, with an expanding array of diagnoses and drugs, that have become slicker, more aggressive, more dangerous, and even more dishonest. Returning to Healy's latest book, he explains how this was done to promote Prozac:

> *The Prozac story is one of a wholesale creation of depression on so extraordinary and unwarranted a scale as to raise grave questions about whether pharmaceutical and other health care companies are more wedded to making profits from health than contributing to it.*

*Not only was depression aggressively promoted to create a
thriving market for Prozac, it was promoted despite troubling
results during its clinical trials in 1987, including suicides,
serious side effects, and subjects dropping out of the studies
rather than continuing to experience drug-induced distress (see
Chapter 8 for details), that, if shared with the public, would
have severely limited its prospects. It is particularly disturbing
that Eli Lilly, the manufacturer, went on to promote the drug
for use in children with full knowledge of these facts.*

Why are dangerous drugs allowed into the marketplace? Pharmaceutical companies control the flow of information to the extent
that they can tilt decision-making so that substances with no proven
benefits, yet significant risks, are allowed on the market, to be dis-
pensed by physicians operating with misleading and incomplete
information.

To begin with, the FDA allows researchers connected to
pharmaceutical companies, who have a financial stake in the
outcome, to be members of drug approval advisory panels (often
making up 50% of the members). [5]

And the evidence these panels are reviewing? It comes from
studies conducted by the drug companies themselves, where positive results are reported an unsurprising 98% of the time. Are the
drugs really this good? Of course not, but their creators are very
good at suppressing negative outcomes and massaging positive
outcomes. So why doesn't the government demand that negative
results get released along with the positive? The studies are proprietary, which means they are the property of the pharmaceutical companies who fund them and are not obligated to make the
results public.

Think about it: pharmaceutical companies conduct the
bulk of the research on psychiatric drugs, and, not only do they
get to ignore people who died or dropped out of clinical trials
due to severe side effects in estimating risk, they can bury studies that do not give them the answers they want. Just having
firms with a huge financial interest being trusted with any kind
of studies that will be relied upon in the FDA approval process

is worrisome, but that they can pick and choose what is evaluated, with rarely any suitable alternative sources of information to be drawn on, is frightening.

Not only do pharmaceutical companies get to doctor the flow of information, but they also have a hand in determining treatment guidelines for the unproven psychiatric diseases they helped create, which includes, of course, directions for administering the medications they make billions of dollars from. Surveys have revealed that 9 of 10 medical experts responsible for writing treatment guidelines have financial ties to the pharmaceutical industry, though these are rarely revealed. Is it any wonder, then, that anybody who looks at the criteria for psychiatric disorders can always find a varied assortment they qualify for, along with a supermarket size selection of drugs to treat them? The intent is to cast as wide a net as possible—and fill the mouths of those caught in it with every profitable substance possible.

The precedent for the practice of creating a disease as a means of manufacturing demand for a psychiatric drug got its start with Ritalin and its amphetamine cousins. As we showed earlier, it was only after the drug had been found to improve focus and manageability in children did the ADD/ADHD diagnoses appear and quickly begin evolving to include growing numbers of children. With huge profits being made, Ritalin was ripe for challengers. And who conquered it in terms of market share? A drug already deemed too dangerous for adults.

It hit the scene in a big way during the mid-90s, when Shire Pharmaceutical decided to overtake Ritalin with a product of its own and launched a multi-million dollar campaign to promote Adderall, a mix of amphetamine salts that had been a big money maker as a diet drug in years past but was taken off the market in the early 1980s because so many women became addicted to it (as we detailed in chapter two).

Despite its sordid history Adderall, like Dexedrine before it, made a comeback as an ADHD drug, too dangerous for dieting adults but perfectly okay for fidgety kids. Launched in 1996,

Adderall's sales hit $19 million in 1997, $200 million in 2000, and an incredible $400 million, over 40% of company revenues, in 2002. Lightning had struck twice, and this was just for medications aimed at a single disease. How much more money could be made by dusting off other existing drugs and attaching them to diagnoses that could be made to mirror either normal childhood behavior, or, even worse, that of normal kids in the midst of real emotional trauma? Sure enough, what worked for Adderall is now being successfully implemented with a wide range of other adult drugs (like the desipramine that killed Shaina Dunkle) that kids are the targeted recipients of, for a constantly expanding menu of maladies. The danger level has been cranked way up from Ritalin, which is almost starting to look quaint in comparison.

One of the most frightening examples of pharmaceutical company drug pushing came in the May 13, 2004 announcement from the Justice Department that Pfizer had pled guilty to charges that it had wrongly promoted Neurontin, an epilepsy drug, for unapproved uses and agreed to pay $430 million, which included a $240 million criminal fine, the second largest ever in the prosecution of health care fraud. The Justice Department has made settlements for over $2 billion since the year 2000 as the result of investigations into how big pharmaceutical companies market their drugs illegally.

In 2003 Pfizer's revenues were $45.1 billion, and $2.7 billion of that came from sales of Neurontin. The drug was approved in 1993 as an anti-seizure medication for sufferers of epilepsy. Once a drug has been approved by the FDA physicians are free to prescribe it as they see fit, be it for the approved use or not, but pharmaceutical companies are not allowed to promote drugs for off-label use. What the Justice Department's investigation revealed was that Warner-Lambert (a division of Parke-Davis before Pfizer bought it in 2000) blatantly violated the law by marketing Neurontin as a treatment for ADHD, bipolar disorder, Lou Gehrig's disease, migraine headaches, and even restless leg syndrome, among others.

Much like other pharmaceutical companies, they paid physicians to hear presentations on the off-label use of Neurontin under the guise of "consultant meetings," held in places like Hawaii and Florida. Warner-Lambert also employed medical liaisons, who presented themselves to physicians as experts on the different diseases they wanted Neurontin to be used for. There was no evidence of the usefulness or safety of Neurontin for any of these off-label treatments, and patients who took the drug were essentially unknowing subjects in a completely unethical experiment.

It is not much different for that old ADHD standby, Ritalin. As a stimulant it is appropriate for narcolepsy—a real disease— but not for the committee-created ADHD. Ritalin is deemed effective, remember, because, like other stimulants, it enhances the ability of the person who takes it to stay focused on boring tasks, but the fact that a drug achieves a result some people might want, be it because it makes them money or puts "more sheep in the seats," does not mean it is treating a legitimate medical condition. The problem is that pharmaceutical companies have discovered that they do not need proof; all they need to do is create a suitable illusion that appears to come with enough benefits that it will not be looked at too hard.

On June 11, 2003 a joint study done by Harvard and MIT was released that revealed direct-to-consumer advertising by the pharmaceutical industry increased from $800 million in 1996 to $2.7 billion in 2001. Not only that, but with a return on investment of $4.20 in sales for every $1 spent on advertising, we can expect even more in the future. And bear in mind, this blitz is not done to inform consumers, but to misinform them—in hopes they will be worried into scheduling a physician visit, where a busy doctor who is being paid for a 15 minute session, and maybe just as badly informed as the patient, is likely to prescribe a drug as a seemingly efficient means of addressing the presenting problem.

"Welcome to Ordinary" says a full-page advertisement for the antidepressant Strattera, in the September 2003 issue of *Family Circle*, which is being pushed hard for childhood and adult ADHD.

So if a parent reads that, after being convinced that truly ordinary childhood behaviors, that just happen to be annoying or difficult to deal with are evidence of impairment, and decides to bring a child to their pediatrician, how hard can it be to get the drug? They have already been instructed in how to go about it. No wonder annual sales of ADHD drugs have topped $2 billion.

DOCTORED DECEIT

The billions in sales for ADHD drugs, antidepressants, and other psychiatric drugs, could not occur without physicians willingly taking up their pens to write prescriptions. They, unfortunately, are too often just as badly misinformed as parents and patients who are swayed by direct-to-consumer advertisements. On April 22, 2004 the highly respected British medical journal, *The Lancet* [6], published an article that was the first meta-analysis done in a peer-reviewed journal of all available drug trials on a specific group of antidepressants. It was conducted by six British academic psychiatrists and researchers who said that, although some published studies made the newer antidepressants (SSRIs) appear effective to doctors, five studies never made public by the pharmaceutical companies who funded them showed that the benefits (if any) did not justify the risks. The drugs in question are popular antidepressant medications: Paxil (paroxetine), Effexor (venlafaxine), Zoloft (sertraline), and Celexa (citalopram) .

In an editorial [7] in the same issue the journal took the FDA to task for failing to "...act appropriately on information...that these drugs are both ineffective and harmful in children." The editors also wrote:

> *The story of research into selective serotonin reuptake inhibitor [SSRI] use in childhood depression is one of confusion, manipulation, and institutional failure. In a global culture where evidence-based practice is seen as the gold standard for care, these failings are a disaster.*

"Disaster" is a strong word for a top medical journal, but it fits. Earlier in April 2004 another respected publication, *BMJ* (formerly the *British Medical Journal*) expressed the opinion that the drug-company-paid-for studies that were published downplayed the risks of these drugs and overstated their usefulness, saying, "Biased reporting and overconfident recommendations in treatment guidelines may mislead doctors, patients, and families." So deceitful is the process that Dr. Jane Garland of British Columbia's Children's Hospital, where she heads a clinic for mood and anxiety disorders, a physician who has worked in some of the pharmaceutical industry's drugs trials, was reported by the above journal to have pledged, "never to do an industry-funded trial again unless the whole structure and management of these is drastically changed."

The message is clear: The studies published in even the most prestigious medical journals, which physicians have long relied on, are subject to corruption when it comes to psychiatric drugs. They are a biased, deceitful source of information and, sadly, few alternatives exist. The pharmaceutical companies have mostly taken over what used to be mechanisms for the dissemination of objective scientific results. If you are a parent, then, and bring your child to a physician out of concern over a problem you have been told he may need to be given a psychiatric drug for, that physician may be operating under the influence of information of no better quality than the Strattera advertisement in *Family Circle*. Tim Kendall, director of the National Collaborating Centre for Mental Health, located in London, who was one of the authors of the bombshell article in *The Lancet*, was quoted in the April 24, 2004 issue of *The Washington Post* as saying, "In each of the published articles, the authors concluded the drug was either effective or safe or both. When you look at the combined evidence, it is ineffective, unsafe, or both."

Just imagine if pharmaceutical companies were honest about antidepressants (and this would hold true for ADHD drugs and many others, too), what would the result be? Would they make any money? As Kendall also said, "If I wanted to introduce a new drug for children who are suicidal and said this has very little proof of efficacy and it has an increased risk of suicide, people would say I was mad." When it comes to antidepressants for children, then, honesty and sound medical judgment would result in no sales. Deliberate dishonesty and fraud translate into billions of dollars—and millions of abused children.

THE EROSION OF GOVERNMENT PROTECTION

But wait a second, shouldn't the government intervene; shouldn't some official body step in to protect our children? We can call the police if somebody tries to assault or rob them, so surely there's an emergency service available when children are being chemically attacked and robbed of their childhoods, right? No. The pharmaceutical industry is enormously powerful, powerful enough to strongly influence everything from the classification of new psychiatric disorders, medical research, medical training, information given to educators, the position of mental health advocacy groups, and the federal government itself. The following excerpt from the August 26, 2003 issue of the British newspaper, *The Guardian*, states the dilemma clearly:

> *Since the early 1990s, the pharmaceutical industry has been the most profitable industry in America, with margins exceeding 18%. With profit has come power. In the 1999-2000 election cycle, the drug industry spent more money on political lobbying than any other industry, more than the oil and gas industry, more than tobacco, more than the insurance or automobile industry. The drug industry has also ratcheted up its spending on doctors. The number of drug representatives employed to make pitches directly to doctors rose by 57% in the 1990s to a total of 88,000 by the end of the decade. Perhaps most remarkably, the drug industry now funds 40% of continuing education in American medical schools.*

Not only do pharmaceutical companies spend more on lobbying than any other industry, they also employ more lobbyists, with the total exceeding the total number of people serving in the House of Representatives. They also fund mental health advocacy, support, and educational groups, pay for the continuing education of physicians, and contribute heavily to all manner of public awareness efforts. In short, it is difficult to find a single area of discourse on the issue of psychiatric drugs and diagnoses that they are not involved in or influencing. Never before has an industry held this kind of sway over public and professional consciousness.

What happens when a member of the "establishment" steps up and challenges this bankrolled consciousness? Most often they are ignored, ridiculed, or silenced. For example, in 2003 the FDA assigned their leading expert, Dr. Andrew Mosholder, the task of investigating the emerging (though it had been around for years) evidence of a link between antidepressants and suicide attempts in children. As he was told to, he did his job and filed his report, but the FDA refused to release it. They also refused to allow him to participate in public hearings on antidepressants that were conducted in February 2004. Why? Our belief is that it is because of his finding that children who take antidepressants are two times more likely to exhibit suicidal behaviors than depressed children who are not given antidepressants. Indeed, in March of 2004, when the FDA issued a warning on antidepressant use in children, it made no mention that their top expert had gone through the results of 28 clinical trials funded by the pharmaceutical companies who make the antidepressants in questions—and most of these studies had been withheld from the public and medical professionals, especially those sporting negative results.

Dr. Mosholder's report, as of this writing, still remains buried, but news of its contents made it into a CBS News report and his findings were shared by the *Los Angeles Times* by way of an internal FDA document they obtained. A sentence by Mosholder in it addressed limitations in the data and read, "Finding a statistical association despite these limitations makes the finding difficult to dismiss." Unfortunately, it will be eagerly dismissed by those with a financial and/or professional interest in believing otherwise. Quoted in the April 6, 2004 *Los Angeles Times*, Harvard psychiatrist Dr. Joseph Glenmullen said, "Evidence that they're suppressing a report like this is an outrage, given the public health and safety issues at stake."

SMOKE AND MIRRORS

One of the favorite tactics of those who promote invented diseases and ineffective, dangerous drugs is taking unsupported assumptions and weak correlations and presenting them as root causes. For example, functional brain scans (those which show the different 'set' of the brain corresponding to different moods) show the brains of depressed people to look different than those who are not depressed, a finding used to justify the belief that it too is a disease. Yet all this finding does is provide evidence of a correlation between biological dynamics and what is categorized as depression. Because the brain is a living organ constantly responding to its environment with complex neurochemical and electrical changes, it is most likely that the biological dynamics are a result of the interplay of emotions, thoughts, intentions, and behaviors seen in people diagnosed as depressed. Be it by genetics, temperament, or environmental circumstance some people may be more prone to depression than others, but the best review of the evidence [8] concluded that "...the neuroimaging literature provides no convincing evidence for the existence of abnormality in the brains of depressed persons." Nor is there any for children said to be suffering from anxiety disorders, ADHD, bipolar, oppositional defiant disorder, and on and on down the list of imaginary diseases.

What are diagnosed as psychiatric disorders are most often the result of some kind of stress, and the kinds of stress children are subject to is well documented, be it the myriad types of dysfunction at home (divorce, abuse, alcoholism, lack of parental attention, etc.), unyielding school systems that refuse to tolerate or acknowledge the diversity of human temperament, abilities, interests, and learning styles, or simply living in an uncertain world that grows more threatening and complex.

Okay, but even so, shouldn't we go ahead and medicate kids with psychological problems, regardless of the cause?

They are easy to administer, take little time and effort, cost insurance companies less money, and don't require anybody to really get to know a child well enough to figure out what's bothering her and what to do about it. Naturally, pharmaceutical companies spend billions to convince parents, educators, and health care professionals that the drugs are superior. Why talk to children about their problems when drugs will damp down the symptoms?

An adult can say no to a drug that is hurting her and walk away. A child is powerless to resist and likely to have the ill effects of one drug treated by adding others to the mix, which only compounds the problem. If so many adults died from Prozac during a supervised trial, what will the death toll climb to in children whose systems are so much more sensitive? We are already witnessing a rapidly mounting body count, and, just because a child appears okay, for now, on an adult drug, developing brains are far more vulnerable than adult brains and brain damage generally becomes more apparent after the brain is fully developed.

Targeting a powerless group for abuse under cover of medical diagnoses is not new, even in the United States. It happened during slavery when rebellious slaves were diagnosed with conditions that purported to explain their bad behavior and provided excuses for punishing it. In a chilling preview of today's attention deficit, oppositional defiant conduct, and borderline personality disorders we so love to brand children with, Dr. Samuel Cartwright, a 19th century physician, came up with the label "Drapetomania," a condition that, "manifests itself by an irresistible propensity to run away," and "Dysoesthesia oethiopeca," which described a diseased slave as "paying no attention to the rights of property," and "breaking the tools he works with," and engaging in "idleness and sloth." Though there are plenty of exceptions where psychiatry is genuinely used in a child's best interest, we are faced with millions of diagnoses of children that have no more scientific basis than did those applied to slaves, and both serve the same purpose, the justification of abuse and oppression.

In recent years the practice of dispensing drugs for bogus diagnoses has made another distressing step. Now, when one drug is given and the symptoms worsen, instead of taking the child off the drug, other drugs are added. So not only are children put on drugs that should never be found in their bodies, the new push is to give them more when the original do not work. Too many are still inclined to believe what psychiatry says of the safety and efficacy of the drugs it tests, not stopping to consider that their every disorder/disease is a fraud. I am of the opinion that their entire literature is bought and paid for and is not to be believed.

It started when children who had adverse reactions to the stimulants they were given for ADHD were said to have additional disorders and to need other drugs to counter the ill effects. Rarely was it considered that the ADHD drugs themselves might be the problem, so adult drugs were added to counter the new problems of sleeplessness, depression, anxiety, delusions, and hallucinations that are sure to result when so many children are given drugs essentially the same as cocaine and speed.

Prescribing drugs approved for adults but never tested in children, or approved for use in that population, is the off-label prescribing Pfizer got in trouble for with for Neurontin. It seems that pharmaceutical companies can promote the practice without leaving behind the kind of trail that lands them in court. So, if a child has mood swings from the Adderall (which isn't surprising with an amphetamine cocktail) he is on, why not add the adult diagnosis of bipolar disorder and treat it with adult drugs like Depakote (primarily an anticonvulsant drug)? If a child becomes agitated and cannot sleep or eat when her Ritalin prescription goes up why not diagnose an anxiety disorder and bring Paxil into the mix? Rarely do physicians consider that the Ritalin, that cocaine cousin, could be the problem. And if a child starts acting violent or psychotic? Well, there's always the heavy psychiatric artillery, like Haldol, Risperdal and Thorazine.

Today, ADHD is no longer necessary to start the diagnosing and drugging process. Anxiety, borderline personality, bipolar, and all the other disorders can be gone to immediately, along with the drugs that accompany them. Before long the total number of kids branded with these conditions will eclipse the 6 million American children diagnosed with ADHD. And all of it will be supported with a multi-billion dollar edifice constructed by pharmaceutical companies in collusion with schools, psychiatrists, and anybody else who benefits from the linguistic and chemical abuse of children.

PET SCAN "PROOF" –ZAMETKIN, 1990

In the early nineties the APA and NIMH—invested all of their hopes and press releases in the never-replicated, never-confirmed, PET scan study of Zametkin, et al. [9], which—no surprise—turned out to be a powerful illusion of a disease. In their 1994 book, *Driven to Distraction*, psychiatrists Edward Hallowell and John Ratey wrote: "What Zametkin found using this technique was a deficit in glucose uptake, and hence energy use in the brains of subjects with ADD... Zametkin and his colleagues at the National Institutes of Mental Health may not have defined how it happened, but they did demonstrate for sure that it was happening, that the biochemical dance was different in the brains of people with ADD as compared to the brains of people without it." Despite the fact that the Zametkin research, like all research in psychiatry ultimately failed to prove that ADHD was a disease or anything at all, medical or biological, this study and its spurious publicity in the hands of organized psychiatry lead, as nothing else, to the burgeoning of the ADHD epidemic from approximately one million in 1990 to 4.4 million in 1998. As we shall see, time and again, the failure to prove that ADHD is a disease, has never lead to its "cure" or an end to the "epidemic."

GENETIC CAUSES? DO THEY EXIST AT ALL?

Psychiatric researchers forever claim that an abnormal gene or genes (abnormal genotype) is the cause of ADHD and all of their never-proved "diseases"/ "chemical imbalances." Never having proved them to be diseases (abnormality = disease) how can they seek their causes (cause = etiology)? In medicine, the disease is discovered, following which, its cause or causes are sought. In 1972, I discovered and described CHANDS—the Curly Hair-Ankyloblepharon-Nail Dysplasia Syndrome (abnormality = disease = abnormal phenotype), following which, in 1979, Toriello, Lindstrom, Waterman and Baughman elucidated and described its abnormal genotype. (see Chapter 4). Likewise, the acquired immunodeficiency syndrome (AIDS) was encountered before the human immunodeficiency virus (HIV), was proven to be the cause. Researches are familiar with phenylketonuria due to an absence or marked diminution of the enzyme phenylalanine hydroxylase (with a resultant build-up of phenylalanine and deficiency of tyrosine) due to an absent or defective autosomal recessive gene—the PKU genotype. If there is no physical trait or abnormality, i.e., abnormal phenotype there is no physical manifestation of a particular genotype. Such is a persistent problem with ADHD and all of biological psychiatry where they continually claim the presence of abnormal genes-genotypes as the cause of psychiatric disorders, where they have yet to confirm the presence of a single physical abnormality/disease/abnormal phenotype. Psychiatry's reason for talking, writing, researching and practicing as though theirs was a biological, medical field is to create illusions of "chemical imbalances"/ "diseases" which, they hope, will justify the "chemical balancers"/ drugs! It is a no less diabolical sham.

IF NOT PET SCANS, PERHAPS MRI IS WORTH A TRY

When nothing else panned out, ADHD researchers recalled that in 1986, Nasrallah [11] had produced brain atrophy/shrinkage/shriveling merely by "treating" hyperactive/ADD/ADHD subjects with the usual amphetamines and amphetamine-like drugs. "That's it! We'll treat them, cause brain atrophy, and say ADHD did it. And that's exactly what they have done with their anatomic-structural Magnetic Resonance Imaging (MRI) brain scan research from 1986 to the present time. [10]

On May 13, 1998, F. Xavier Castellanos of the NIMH confessed to me (FB) in a letter, "...we have not yet met the burden of demonstrating the specific pathophysiology that we believe underlies this condition." He was responding to a letter of mine where I asked him for proof that ADHD was a real disease. This was one of but a few truthful statements I have extracted from the leaders of psychiatry in a decade of putting the disease/no disease question to them. "We believe" he said, and that was their justification for "treating" the 4 million already diagnosed.

Nasrallah, et al. (1986) [11] did structural- anatomic- computerized tomographic (CT) brain scans on twenty-four males with a childhood history of hyperkinesis/minimal brain dysfunction (HK/MBD—forerunner of ADHD), all treated with stimulant drugs during childhood. Fifty-eight percent (58%), fourteen of twenty-four, had brain atrophy, compared to one of twenty-seven, controls (3.8 percent). They concluded: "... since all of the HK/MBD patients had been treated with psychostimulants, cortical atrophy may be a long-term adverse effect of this treatment."

With this finding, Nasrallah et al., challenged the ADHD research community to compare ADHD-untreated subjects to ADHD-treated subjects to determine if the brain atrophy in their study was a function of the never validated "disease"—ADHD, or of the Ritalin/amphetamine treatment. All it would take to make HK/MBD/ADD/ADHD a disease would be to find an abnormality, and this had never been done before they changed the definition—diagnostic criteria—and moved on with their diagnosing. If the ADHD subjects are treated, whether with one or several drugs—the treatment, being a known physical factor—would be the only likely cause of any abnormality found.

To tell whether ADHD or a drug is causing a given abnormality one would have to compare (a) ADHD-treated to (b) ADHD-untreated. If only (a) the ADHD-treated are found to be abnormal, not (b) ADHD-untreated, it would have to be concluded that the treatment—the drug or drugs—is the cause of the abnormality.

Now, let us look at the structural-anatomic CT and MRI brain scan research from Nasrallah et al. in 1986 through the ADHD Consensus Conference, held at the National Institutes of Health, November 16-18, 1998.

SWANSON & CASTELLANOS DECLARE ADHD A DISEASE

At the ADHD Consensus Conference (1998), James M. Swanson and F. Xavier Castellanos [12] reviewed the structural-anatomic MRI scan literature, the only evidence, they claimed, suggesting that ADHD was an actual disease, a brain disease. They concluded: "Recent investigations provide converging evidence that a refined phenotype of ADHD/HKD is characterized by reduced size in specific neuroanatomical regions of the frontal lobes and basal ganglia." Nor did they (Swanson presenting) leave any doubt that they were claiming that the brain atrophy was due to ADHD and was the long-sought, biological basis of ADHD.

The 14 such studies Swanson and Castellanos reviewed at the Consensus Conference [Hynd et al. (1990)[13], Hynd et al. (1991)[14], Hynd et al. (1993)[15], Giedd et al. (1994) [16], Castellanos et al. (1994)[17] Semrud-Clikeman et al. (1994)[18], Baumgardner et al. (1996)[19], Aylward et al. (1996)[20], Castellanos et al. (1996)[21], Filipek et al. (1997)[22], Casey et al. (1997)[23], Mataro et al. (1997)[24], Berquin et al. (1998)[25], and Mostofsky

et al. (1998)[26] all scanned ADHD-treated subjects—never an
ADHD untreated group-proving, time and again, that the treat-
ment/drugs, not the never-validated "disease" ADHD, was the
cause of the brain atrophy. Two of these studies did not report
whether the ADHD subjects were medicated or not, and one did
not report clearly. Leo and Cohen [27] estimate that 247 of the 259
total ADHD subjects in these studies [13-26]—95%—had been
medicated ("ADHD-medicated").

Nonetheless, in virtually all of these studies, the titles, ab-
stracts, conclusions, and press releases, crowed the finding of
brain atrophy/shrinkage and insisted, time and again, that this
was the proof that ADHD is a brain disease. Not a word was said
of the fact that virtually all of the subjects were "treated" with the
toxins—Ritalin and a variety of amphetamines, or that they, not
the never-validated "disease" ADHD, was the probable cause of
their brain atrophy.

When Swanson had finished his Consensus Conference presentation, not saying a word about the "treated" status of virtually all of the ADHD subjects in the studies reviewed, I took a
floor microphone and asked: "Dr. Swanson, why didn't you mention that virtually all of the ADHD subjects in the neuroimaging
studies have been on chronic stimulant therapy and that this is
the likely cause of their brain atrophy?" Swanson: "This is a critical issue and in fact I am planning a study to investigate that."
Here we had a confession from leading ADHD researcher, James
M. Swanson, that all of the CT and MRI scan research from that
of Narallah in 1986, through the Consensus Conference in 1998,
had been done carried out on ADHD "treated"/ Ritalin/amphet-
amine-exposed subjects, while none at all had been carried out on
untreated groups with ADHD!

Had their intention, all these years been to find out what
the brains of ADHD (untreated) children looked like? Or, was
it with *knowledge of the Nasrallah study of 1986* that treatment
with Ritalin and the amphetamines was the likely cause of the
brain atrophy, that they (all ADHD brain scan researchers) in-

tended to replicate that study, time and again, and portray the resultant brain atrophy/shrinkage, not as due to the drugs, but as the "proof" that ADHD is a disease—proof they never had, proof they needed to justify the continued prescribing of billions of dollars worth of Ritalin and amphetamine "treatments" to children who were, in fact, entirely normal until their "treatment" began.

With no proof of a biological basis for ADHD, the final statement of the Consensus Conference Panel, could only be: "...we do not have an independent, valid test for ADHD, and there are no data to indicate that ADHD is due to brain malfunction" [27] [28]. This was a confession that there was no proof that ADHD was a disease. As we have seen above, the Panel should have confessed much more, but didn't. [I recommend the video, *ADHD-Total, 100% Fraud*, available at www.adhdfraud.com which shows all of the aforementioned "experts" on the official Consensus Conference videotape trying their best, with very little success, to justify the drugging of millions of our entirely normal children.]

From a January, 2000, *Readers Digest* article [29]: "Castellanos and his group found three areas of the brain to be significantly smaller in ADHD kids than in normal children... Some critics claim that such brain differences in ADHD children might actually be caused by Ritalin...To address this, Castellanos has now embarked on another study, imaging the brains of ADHD youngsters who have not been treated with drugs. Two years post-Consensus Conference and Castellanos is just now embarking on a study to image the brains of ADHD youngsters who have not been treated with drugs."

* * *

In 2001, Baumeister and Hawkins [8] wrote: "Neuroimaging studies have been conducted with increasing frequency in recent years in attempts to identify structural and functional abnormalities in the brains of persons with attention deficit/hyperactivity disorder. Although the results of these studies are frequently cited in support of a biologic etiology for this disorder, inconsistencies among studies raise questions about the reliability of the findings. The present review (theirs) shows that no specific abnormality in brain structure or function has been convincingly demonstrated by neuroimaging studies."

Thirty-five years of representing ADHD and other psychiatric conditions to be diseases, and still no proof! Regardless of age, those said to have psychiatric "diseases"/ "chemical imbalances" and drugged, are medically/biologically normal until drugged/poisoned—always with their right to informed consent having been abrogated.

STILL REFUSING TO DO VALID RESEARCH

On October 9, 2002, Castellanos et al. [30] reported: "...the first neuroimaging study (the first in all of the MRI literature, 1986-2002) to our knowledge to include a substantial number (n=49) of previously unmedicated children and adolescents with ADHD." Here we have a confession there has never in 16 years of brain scanning been a study of an ADHD-unmedicated group of patients. The 49 ADHD-unmedicated subjects had a mean age of 8.3 years vs. the 139 controls with whom they were compared, with a mean age of 10.5 years; 2.2 years younger! How could the ADHD-unmedicated subjects not be smaller, overall? How could they not have smaller bodies, heads, brains? Next, they compared ADHD-medicated (n=103) to ADHD-unmedicated (n=49) subjects. The ADHD-unmedicated subjects, mean age 8.3 years, were 2.6 years younger than the ADHD-medicated subjects, mean age 10.9 years. Nor were these two groups suitable for comparison. But this did not stop Castellanos, et al. from concluding, as it was predetermined that they should, that: (1) "...the cerebrum as a whole and the cerebellum (essentially, the whole brain) are smaller in children and adolescents with predominantly combined type ADHD," and (2) "Conversely, we have no evidence that stimulant drugs cause abnormal brain development." Neither conclusion was justified given that none of the comparisons were valid.

Once again, as throughout 16 years of MRI brain scanning research, Castellanos and the NIMH refused to do a valid study, the comparison of a group of ADHD-untreated to a truly matched group of normal controls. A truly matched control group could have been constituted, but was not. Rather, since the 1986 Nasrallah study, they have known that Ritalin-amphetamine treatment induces brain atrophy and have proven this time-after-time, obscuring however possible their "treated"/"drugged" status while consistently representing that the atrophy produced is, instead, due to ADHD, the abnormality of the brain confirming it is a disease, a brain disease.

Starting with an always-subjective behavioral-emotional, DSM construct, their biological-medical research is destined never to prove a thing. Instead, in this study and in all such studies in "biological psychiatry" the only abnormalities found—and they are real—are those induced by the brain-damaging drugs they are invariably put on.

In fact the entire ADHD-MRI literature, all of it showing atrophy of the brain and brain parts, all of it performed on stimulant-treated subjects is proof, replicated time and again, that these medications, not the never-validated "brain disease" ADHD, are the cause of the brain atrophy.

Using anatomic-structural magnetic resonance imaging (MRI), Bartzokis et al. (2003) [31] found that both cocaine-dependent and amphetamine-dependent adults had significantly smaller temporal lobe volumes (these were not ADHD subjects). This too supports the suspicion that it is the encephalopathic Ritalin/amphetamine drugs that are the cause of the brain atrophy disclosed time and again in the ADHD research of 1986 through the present.

The 2003 study of Sowell et al. [32] showed brain atrophy but once again failed to include an ADHD-untreated group. Can there be any doubt that the their market plan is to scan ADHD-treated subjects, knowing they will find brain atrophy, say little or nothing about the fact of their treatment and then represent, in all but the finest print, the brain atrophy to be the "proof " that ADHD is a "disease."

The 2003 review of Leo and Cohen [33] lead them to conclude: "We found that most subjects diagnosed with ADD or ADHD had prior medication use, often for several months or years. This substantial confound invalidates any suggestion of ADHD-specific neuropathology. Moreover, the few recent studies using unmedicated subjects have inexplicably avoided making straightforward comparisons of these subjects with controls."

In other words they have purposely avoided doing valid scientific research. Why? When will they be held accountable for their deception and the poisoning of millions of normal children?

A CONFESSION: NO SUCH THING AS A PSYCHIATRIC DISEASE

Actually, the answer to the psychiatric disease/no disease question was delivered by Swanson himself on March 7, 1998, in an address to the American Society of Adolescent Psychiatry in San Diego (I was there). He confessed, "I would like to have an objective diagnosis for the disorder (ADHD). Right now psychiatric diagnosis is completely subjective...We would like to have biological tests—a dream of psychiatry for many years." Swanson's saying this means there is no such thing as an actual disease or physical abnormality in all of psychiatry; it means the brain atrophy in all of the studies, from that of Nasrallah, et al. in 1986, up to and including that of Castellanos, et al. in *JAMA*, October 9, 2002 could only be due to their Ritalin/amphetamine therapy; it means that every physical consequence or side effect of every psychiatric "disease" can only be due to the drug treatments themselves, there being no such thing as an actual, real, genuine, bona fide, psychiatric disease.

Swanson's saying this also means that the 6 million children in the US with ADHD were entirely normal until the moment their Ritalin/amphetamine "treatment" was begun.

SPINNING A WEB OF DECEIT

By having so much influence over sources of information and decision-making power, pharmaceutical companies and those who collude with them (the psychiatric and educational establishments in particular) shape consciousness to the point where opinions, assumptions, misinformation, and outright lies are regarded as an accepted body of truth. Once this happens on a large enough scale, it is very difficult to turn the momentum the other way, which is precisely why so many resources are poured into the deceit. For example, though it never had any evidence to back it up and has been proven wrong over and over again, there is still a widespread notion that drugs like Ritalin have a paradoxical effect on ADHD sufferers, meaning these stimulants cause victims of the "disease" to focus and behave better, contrary to what one might think a stimulant does. The truth, of course, is that stimulants have the same effect on everybody. But, the wrongheaded notion sticks, and is still used as a "See, I told you so" when a targeted child "behaves" after being given the drug; the normal response of a normal child is interpreted as evidence of neurological impairment. And this is but one example of a widespread practice.

To close this chapter we will leave you with a passage from Leo Tolstoy that beautifully sums up the problem:

> *I know that most men, including those at ease with problems of the greatest complexity, can seldom accept even the simplest and most obvious truth if it be such as would oblige them to admit the falsity of conclusions which they have delighted in explaining to colleagues, which they have proudly taught to others, and which they have woven, thread by thread, into the fabric of their lives.*

LYING TO PATIENTS–THE NEW STANDARD
OF PRACTICE

On May 28, 2002, I wrote to Bernard Alpert, MD, President of the Medical Board of California (MBC): "Every time parents or a patient is led to believe that their child's emotional/behavioral problem is a "disease" due to an abnormality within their body or brain, they have been lied to, their informed consent rights wholly violated…"

On June 14, 2002, Dr. Alpert, responded: "As you outline in your letter, there is tremendous professional support for categorizing emotional and psychological conditions as diseases of the brain. In published materials, some quoted in your letter, you will find that support from chairs of psychiatry departments, the American Psychiatric Association, and professors of major medical schools. It is clear that the psychiatric community has set their standard, and while one might disagree with it, that standard becomes the legal standard upon which the Board must base its actions."

Unbelievably, what Alpert, speaking for the Medical Board of the State of California is saying here, is that whatever the majority do, even lie, knowingly violating the informed consent rights of all patients, that that becomes the unassailable, legal "standard of practice." Consider, if you will that, conversely, to tell patients the truth—specifically, that ADHD and all psychiatric diseases are not diseases at all, or to fail to prescribe "chemical balancers"—drugs for each and every "chemical imbalance of the brain"—would be contrary to the "standard of practice" putting the physician who is the purveyor of truth and science, in legal jeopardy.

I say to the Congress and now, to President Bush, as well: should you pass any law, in any way, "assuring" or sanctioning the "diagnosis" and "treatment" of psychiatric "diseases"/ "chemical imbalances" in NORMAL children (as is done nation-wide), or should you fail to expunge such laws already on the books—you will have been a party to a fraud.

Chapter Eight

PUSHING POISONS

You have an obligation today to prevent this tragic story from being repeated over and over again.

—Mark Miller, father of Matt Miller, who hung himself after taking seven Zoloft tablets, testifying at the Food and Drug Administration's hearing on antidepressants on February 2, 2004

I t should be clear by now that until an abnormality has been found a disease cannot be diagnosed (abnormality = disease) and medical treatment cannot be justified. This is why no normal child should be "diagnosed" or "treated" and why the millions of children in the US and around the world treated for illusory, psychiatric diseases must be weaned from these poisons, their only chance for resumption of a normal life.

In this chapter more will be said of the dangers of the more common psychotropic drugs given to children in the name of "help" and "treatment."

There is no drug that improves on the normal functioning of the human brain. Though stimulants like Ritalin and Adderall may initially appear to in their capacity to increase focus, this is accomplished by actually damaging the normal brain and is never justifiable. Every drug has some degree of toxicity, and this must be balanced against the benefits provided. In the case of ADHD and all psychiatric disorders, no disease exists and the children so labeled can, therefore, only be considered normal. Being normal, no psychiatric drug is going to improve their brains' functioning and no toxic effects, or the risk of them, can be justified.

The psychological, psychiatric disturbances of children arise from stresses of their environment, be it from their home, school, or community, in other words, in situations controlled by the adults in their lives. When a child is anxious, depressed, or distracted, they are responding to something that is troubling them. Such emotions are a normal barometer of what is happening in the life of the child, a barometer the adults in their lives are obligated to read, understand, and respond to, not drug, mask, and ignore. Maybe a medication can lessen their emotional pain and acting out, but it does not address the child's stress or its causes. In fact, by introducing a toxic substance into a child's body and brain, it is certain her ability to adapt and prevail will be impaired.

Though we talk over and over again about how psychiatric diagnoses in children are not legitimate diseases, syndromes, conditions, or disorders in medical terms, this is not to downplay their seriousness or the pain of emotional suffering. Indeed, far too many children are living in situations that could easily be viewed as worse than most purely physical problems. And this is why it is so important to listen and pay attention to what is really going on, rather than insult our children by claiming their means of expressing themselves are symptoms of diseases that reside within them, and not us, the adults who control their environments.

When it comes to the long term effects of drugs, psychotropic or otherwise, industry drug trials tell us little or nothing, for they usually last just 3-6 weeks and are designed to paint a rosy picture. Deaths may occur, but such facts rarely get into the drug "insert" that is supposed to be all the patient and family need to know to give informed consent to treat. Rather it is the horror stories that slowly emerge in the press from the "post-marketing" prescription experience that are the facts which should constitute "disclosure" for purposes of informed consent, but never do.

Rezulin, a diabetes drug, caused 61 deaths before it was taken off of the market. It took an FDA physician going direct to Congress to get the FDA to act. [1]

Within the short space of 9 months, three FDA-approved drugs have had to be removed from the market due to lethal side effects, that became known, not during pre-marketing safety and efficacy trials, but very soon into their post-marketing, prescription use. Only three times in the past decade has the FDA removed previously approved drugs due to adverse post clinical trials, post-marketing experience. The FDA's approval of drugs that later turned out to have lethal side effects is the predictable result of an industry campaign to speed up the approval process. [2]

It is probably easier to get a feel for the long term effects of training children to believe that they are in the grips of brain diseases and in need of chemical assistance, probably for life, by giving them the message that childhood itself is a disease and that acting as children do, particularly when under stress, is not acceptable. And what of the effects of training children to think that the distress they experience in their lives is an outgrowth of their imbalanced brains, with adults having no responsibility, beyond labeling and medicating them for convenience and profit?

Between there being no formal mechanism for collecting data on adverse reactions to psychiatric drugs among children and the proclivity of pharmaceutical companies to settle lawsuits out of court, on condition the aggrieved parties remain silent, solid numbers on the negative consequences of these drugs are impossible to come by. As for the long-term effects, we are completely in the dark.

On February 2, 2004 the Food and Drug Administration heard testimony on the dangers of antidepressants. A physician who testified, Dr. Lawrence Diller, later spoke of his testimony in an article that appeared in the February 4, 2004 *Christian Science Monitor*, addressing his "loss of faith in my academic colleagues to generate accurate information and opinions that I feel I can trust because of the extremely intimate link between researchers and the drug industry." And what of improving regulation of the medical profession? Diller says this in the same article:

We don't have to worry about regulation of doctors because the government has been bought off and so has the public by the drug industry. The ads directed to consumers convince everyone that life is simply...neurotransmitter bubbles going from one set of synapses to another. The lobbying of the drug industry is legendary—and this is a doctor speaking.

Dr. Diller testified at a hearing where the FDA was gathering information on the risks antidepressants pose to children. With all the antidepressants being questioned both in the United States and in England, one, Prozac, keeps coming up as the sole antidepressant that has been shown to be effective in children. But this drug, in truth, has been very well-documented as a dangerous substance and no benefits to children have ever been objectively (independent of a manufacturer with a financial interest) shown to exist. If Prozac is the "good guy," the others (other SSRIs, Paxil, Zoloft, Celexa, Lexapro) must be pure villainy!

How bad is this one antidepressant the FDA has approved for use in children? Documents obtained under the Freedom of Information Act reveal that two months before Prozac was approved for use in adults in 1987 there had already been 27 deaths during the clinical trials alone—and the first prescription had not even been written yet! 15 deaths were by suicide, 6 by overdose, 4 by gunshot, and 2 by drowning. All were confirmed to be directly related to Prozac. An additional 12 deaths were reported but could not be linked to Prozac with absolute certainty.

So frequent, adverse, and intolerable are the side effects of Prozac, Paxil, Zoloft and the others in the SSRI family of antidepressants, that it is the norm for 15-20% of the people who participate in the clinical trials conducted prior to FDA approval to drop out. Another 10% suffer signs of neurological impairment, including tremors, twitches, and tics.

Britain's Medicines and Healthcare Products Regulatory Agency [3] recently warned physicians against prescribing any SSRI antidepressant except Prozac for youths. No parent knowing all of this about the SSRI antidepressants, would likely give informed consent to treat with such a drug, certainly not after being reminded that depression is not a disease, that all children called depressed, are normal.

None of the people who die or drop out of the clinical trials are included when final estimates are made of a drug's effectiveness or safety, and the pharmaceutical companies who finance the testing do not let physicians or consumers know just how dangerous their wares have clearly proven to be.

If such high percentages of adults cannot tolerate these drugs for even short periods of time, how much higher is the percentage of children taking them who experience harmful side effects? How many children feel like 16-year-old Morgan, who says of the first night he was on Effexor (venlafaxine, structurally novel not related to SSRIs or any other type of antidepressant), "I thought I was going crazy," and that, "I couldn't sleep but I didn't want to stay awake because of the nightmare that I was living. The only option seemed for me to end my life." Morgan lived, though he still suffers drug-induced flashbacks. Other children under the influence of similar drugs feel compelled to act out against others, like the high school student on Prozac who says, "I imagined myself going into the kitchen, grabbing a knife and stabbing my mother." Prior to Prozac he'd never experienced such thoughts. Fortunately for his mother, he did not act on the urge.

Kara Baker was not so fortunate. Thirty-six hours after her mother stopped giving her the Paxil that had been destroying her mentally and physically for the past year, she died from the effects of attempting to withdraw from it. Nobody had told them that Paxil is an addictive drug with sometimes awful consequences for those who attempt to go off it cold turkey. Kara's mother is suing the manufacturer. And there have been plenty of other lawsuits, too, but so wealthy are the pharmaceutical companies that they can afford to settle for millions out-of-court on the condition the claimants remain silent, and are therefore not hindering the generation of billions more in drug sales.

Among the many problems with the psychiatric drugs children are being flooded with, parents and professionals are told the substances are either safe or come with only mild risks, risks that pale next to the horrible future they head off. Only later do we discover they are not so benign. Only later do we discover that, as has been clearly shown with Ritalin and all the other ADHD drugs also, they provide no benefits, educationally or socially, to the children taking them. Without enhancement of the educational outcome there is no justification whatsoever to give them to the physically, medically normal children who are targeted.

Dr. Arthur Caplan, chair of the department of medical ethics at the University of Pennsylvania School of Medicine tells us that, "Any time a child reads a little more slowly, we're talking learning disability and administering Ritalin, or any time a kid acts up a bit, instead of giving him detention, we're drugging him…and I've never met a drug yet, including aspirin, that didn't have some side effects." Ritalin, the first drug to be administered to children *en masse* simply for acting like kids, was presented to parents as the most mild of stimulants, so gentle, in fact, that one couldn't put it in the same category as those nasty amphetamines (which is exactly where the DEA has it). According to the August 27, 2001 *Journal of the American Medical Association* Ritalin is more powerful than cocaine at comparable dosage levels. How far would the Ritalin pushers have gotten if parents we clearly told that from the beginning?

In the spring of 2002 a Yale University study [4] showed that 9 of 10 children who go to see a child psychiatrist will be given a prescription, and most of these prescriptions are for dangerous adult drugs whose effects on children over time nobody knows. At trial the psychiatrist who gave Matthew Miller the Zoloft that killed him estimated that 99% of the drugs he prescribed for children had never been tested in children or approved by the FDA. That means they have never been shown to be safe or effective for his unsuspecting patients, and neither the patients nor parents are ever told. This means there is no scientific basis for such "treatment" and yet it is legal and, in psychiatry, the standard of practice.

At the conclusion of their one appointment Matthew Miller's psychiatrist handed him his first week's supply of Zoloft (all it took to kill him) at no charge, from a stockpile of samples provided by the manufacturer. Does the practice of giving out free "starter kits" sound familiar? It should. Crack dealers do the same thing.

To put the crisis in perspective consider this: between 1990-2000 the Food and Drug Administration received 186 reports of death caused by methylphenidate (Ritalin), the best known of the ADHD drugs, along with 536 reports of other adverse consequences. No wonder the DEA classifies it as a Schedule II drug, along with morphine, opium, and cocaine, the most dangerous and addictive drugs that can be legally prescribed [5] [6]. Is there any doubt that few, if any parents, told of these dangers of Ritalin and the amphetamines and told that ADHD has never been proved to be a disease—that their child is normal—would give "informed consent" to treat.

Taken alone these are shocking statistics. Now consider them again in light of the following statement made by David Kessler in 1992, when he was commissioner of the Food and Drug Administration: "Although the FDA receives many adverse event reports, these probably represent only a fraction of the serious adverse events encountered by providers. Only about one percent of the serious events are reported to the FDA." That is an incredible estimate, only 1 % of the serious adverse events. Think of it, the 186 deaths due to methylphenidate/Ritalin 1990-2000, just 1% of the actual number! But wait, much worse is in store.

During the same 1990-2000 time period the Food and Drug Administration received 2,500 reports of death resulting from Prozac, out of 46,000 total reports of adverse events for the drug. Remember that 1% estimate from Kessler of the FDA above? Remember how Prozac is being touted as the one safe and effective antidepressant for kids? It is unlikely that 250,000 people have died from Prozac, but shouldn't the 2,500 be enough to warn us off giving it to children? Given these facts (all should also look at the fine print 'side effects' in the Prozac insert) and the reality that depression is not a disease, but that all who are depressed are medically and physically normal, no parent should want this drug either for their child, or for themselves.

The World Health Organization reports that Paxil, a drug given to children for anxiety, depression, obsessive-compulsive and bipolar disorder, has the highest incidence of adverse reports, physical and psychological addiction, and severe withdrawal effects of any drug, anywhere, in its class. Why do doctors, then, give it to so many children? Dr. David Healy and a team of researchers from Harvard estimate that Prozac has been responsible for 50,000 deaths around the world since its introduction. Why is that given to anybody?

As bad as such drugs are by themselves, even worse may be in store for children who are given cocktails of them whose ingredients are constantly shifting. A child who is given that stew of amphetamine salts, called Adderall, and has trouble sleeping will probably be given a sleeping pill before being taken off the drug. And if his moods seesaw from the speed saturating his body and brain? Why not diagnose him as bipolar and add Prozac to the mix? And if that messes him up even more? Don't worry, there is still heavier psychiatric artillery—the antipsychotics. Heaven forbid we consider that forcing amphetamines down a child's throat might be the real problem.

Does all of this sound extreme? It should, because it is a very extreme approach to treating children in distress, but that doesn't mean it can't happen—and happen often. Below is the story of a child it almost destroyed.

DANIEL IN THE LION'S DEN

Five-year-old Daniel Rosencranz's kindergarten teacher and the school psychologist insisted he was ADHD and the psychologist even wrote up an evaluation for his mother, Cindy Rosencranz, to give their pediatrician when requesting medication. The pediatrician barely looked at Daniel before prescribing Ritalin. When Cindy brought up the fact that the family had suffered carbon monoxide poisoning two years earlier from a malfunctioning furnace that caused them to be evacuated from their house, the doctor scoffed at the idea such a thing could cause learning difficulties in Daniel.

The first two weeks on medication he was a zombie. Just what they wanted, a quiet, compliant child, but there was no warmth there anymore. No heart. No fire. He didn't even seem like Cindy's son. Another drug, Adderall, was added, then another, Catapres (clonidine). Then Ritalin was discontinued and Wellbutrin (bupropion, another antidepressant never approved by the FDA for use in children) added. Adderall was removed and Zyprexa (a powerful anti-psychotic never tested or approved for use in children either) added. The more medicine they used, the worse he got. He'd be fine for a few weeks, but then it was like uncaging a monster. He started screaming and woke up in the middle of the night hearing voices. Daniel's psychotic episodes began to get more frequent and intense, were brought on by no particular events or circumstances (beside the drugs he was saturated with), and caused him to destroy furniture and try to kill himself and others.

Soon he began a series of stays in psychiatric institutions that lasted until the age of 11. During these years he was put on, and taken off, one drug after another, including those listed above and Tegretol (anticonvulsant), Zoloft (SSRI antidepressant), Risperdal (antipsychotic), Depakote (anticonvulsant), Neurontin (anticonvulsant), and Thorazine (antipsychotic), with none approved by the FDA. Along with ADHD Daniel was diagnosed with bipolar disorder and oppositional defiant disorder. Nobody, not a single psychiatrist, social worker, psychologist, or teacher would listen to Cindy when she said he was not any of these things, but was a child whose brain had been damaged from the carbon monoxide poisoning when he was three.

The psychotic episodes that forced the hospitalizations were due to the multiple drugs he was on—polypharmacy. None of his so-called psychiatric illnesses were real or the cause of the psychosis. During his stays Daniel was sexually abused, physically beaten, forced to wipe himself with a shower curtain, and locked in time-out rooms until he wet his pants, among other things.

Finally, a neurologist confirmed it had been the carbon monoxide poisoning that caused the original learning difficulties, and everything else that followed was the result of medications he never should have been given for imaginary disorders he was never afflicted with.

Eventually Daniel returned home, after losing six years of his life to adult drugs that had no business coursing through his young body and brain. His mother does the best she can to salvage what remains of his childhood.

Not only do they invent diseases out of thin air to have something to "treat," they have no regard whatsoever for real diseases, the victim-in-waiting might have, such as the diffuse encephalopathy (brain damage) from carbon monoxide poisoning that Daniel had. Knowing that Ritalin, Adderall, and a majority of psychiatric drugs worsen seizures, I was constantly chagrined to witness how frequently psychiatrists added such drugs to the anticonvulsants essential for controlling the seizures of epileptic patients. Not only have they come to believe the diagnoses they make are real diseases, they have come to believe that the truckloads of drugs they wield with such élan, are essential.

* * *

In an October 3, 2003, CNN editorial, Lou Dobbs addressed the issue of the epidemic abuse of drugs. Not illegal drugs, but legal substances that are little different in their dangers: "The dramatic increase in the sales of pharmaceuticals not only suggest that Americans are well on their way to becoming depressed, anxiety-ridden and incapable of the focus necessary to understand the world in which we live, but also that we are on our way to becoming a drug-dependent nation...A crisis looms."

Let us do everything in our power to see to it that our children do not end up drug-dependent in the course of trying to negotiate the normal challenges that come with being alive.

THE RIGHT (& DUTY) OF INFORMED CONSENT

The main groups of drugs given to our normal children and the normal children of the world by the legal, licit, pharmaceutical industry are (1) the psychostimulants—Ritalin, Dexedrine, Desoxyn (methamphetamine), Adderall, Cylert, Focalin, Metadate, Concerta, etc. (with the recent addition of Strattera from Eli Lilly; (2) the SSRI antidepressants Prozac, Paxil, Zoloft, Lexapro, Celexa, etc.; (3) the tricyclic and heterocyclic antidepressants Tofranil, Norpramin (desipramine), Elavil, Desyrel, Sinequan, Vivactil, Surmontil etc.; (4) atypical antidepressants—Effexor, Wellbutrin; (5) anticonvulsants (Depakote, Depakene, Tegretol, Neurontin, Topamax, etc.); and (6) antipsychotics (Thorazine, Mellaril, Risperdal, Seroquel, Abilify, Clozapine, Clozaril, Geodon, Haldol, Loxitane, Navane, Orap, Zyprexa, etc.).

Not only is informed consent a right, it should be every person's duty to themselves, their children and parents (when they act for their children, parents or others) to insist on having all the facts they need to make a fully informed decision regarding their treatment. This can be difficult, given proprietary interests and the proprietary mindset that would conceal everything negative, but in the case of psychiatry, informed consent must begin with knowing all that is necessary about the condition which they—psychiatry, government, and the pharmaceutical industry—invariably insist is an abnormality/disease/chemical imbalance of the brain, but which is none of these things. This, when it comes to drug treatment in psychiatry, should be the deal-breaker all by itself, the reason, never to take their drugs or, at least, never to give them to your normal child, or to your normal, aging parent, both of whom would only be worse off for having such foreign compounds/poisons coursing through their brains and bodies. So there you have it: on the risk side of the risk vs. benefit analysis you have no disease at all, an illusion of a disease—a normal child/person.

We have told you more than you need to know to know about the risks of the psychostimulants being absolutely unacceptable—that they are highly addictive, that they cause anger, aggression, violence, psychosis, seizures, involuntary movements, brain shrinkage, stunting of growth, high blood pressure, cardiac arrhythmias, cardiomyopathy and death. Once again, all you have to do is, recall that your child is normal, and read all of the side effects—what they admit to—in the drug insert. You should need no further convincing. In fact, the federal government at large and the FDA in particular should expressly prohibit the prescription use of any drugs whatsoever other than for children with clearly defined, diagnosable, physical abnormalities/diseases.

We have discussed the considerable morbidity and mortality of the SSRI antidepressants (Prozac, Paxil, Zoloft, etc.) and why none of them, Prozac included, should ever be given to normal children regardless of their mood, psychological state or psychiatric disorder—none of which are diseases, none of which have an immutable 'prognosis' as does a disease.

The very same must be concluded about the exceedingly dangerous tricyclic and heterocyclic antidepressants (Tofranil, Norpramin (desipramine), Elavil, Desyrel, etc.). Recall the spate of sudden cardiac deaths reported in the mid-1990s leading psychiatrist John Werry of New Zealand to urge that they be banned from use in children, a suggestion beaten back by friends of industry. Recall the deaths of Cameron Pettus and Shaina Dunkle both from desipramine, a member of this class of antidepressants. These drugs should never be given to children under any circumstances. What adults do when they have had all the facts (which is almost never the case) is up to them.

The risk vs. benefit analysis of (4) atypical antidepressants (Effexor, Wellbutrin) is no different than that for the SSRIs or tri- or hetero-cyclic antidepressants; they should never be given to a normal child, which is to say, any child with an illusory psychiatric disease/chemical imbalance.

The (5) anticonvulsants (Depakote, Depakene, Topamax Tegretol, Neurontin, etc.) as a group are not as dangerous or deadly as any of the drugs of groups 1, 2, 3, 4 and 6, but all are foreign compounds, poisons, and should never be used as mental health treatment in medically normal children. When used to treat the epilepsies (seizure disorders), we have a disease and a diseased, abnormal child on the risk side of the risk/benefit equation, and a scientific rationale and medical justification to treat—something that is never the case in psychiatry.

The (6) antipsychotics (Thorazine, Mellaril, Risperdal, Seroquel, Abilify, Clozapine, Geodon, Clozaril, Haldol, etc.) are such an especially brain- and body-toxic group of drugs, that it should be criminal to give to any normal child. At times I have prescribed anti-psychotic drugs to brain-damaged, retarded, children (clearly abnormal/diseased) who could be controlled no other way. Drugs of this group can induce a Parkinson's syndrome, or dystonias—torticollis and retrocollis (which often abate with cessation of the medication) and tardive (late onset) dyskinesias (involuntary writhing and tic like movements) which are often permanent and untreatable. Other side effects include bulbar paralysis with aspiration and death, weight gain, diabetes, brain atrophy (evident on CT or MRI scan, cardiac arrhythmias (including cardiac arrest and death) and the most feared complication of all, neuroleptic-malignant syndrome (NMS), with which the limbs and body stiffen, the temperature climbs uncontrollably, muscle disintegrates leaking myoglobin into the blood, causing clotting within the vessels, and, shutting down of the kidneys, leading to death. Need we say no drug in this group should every be given to a normal child.

As always, look at the "side effects" in the drug insert. You will find most or all of these side effects mentioned which is industry's way of protecting themselves as they do all they can legally to assure that psychiatrists and as many other physicians as possible will desert what medical science they learned and use all of their products to treat the mental illnesses/disorders/chemical imbalances, industry itself has crafted such indelible illusions of.

GETTING OFF PSYCHIATRIC DRUGS

Clearly, our intention here is to prevent any further drugging of the normal children of this or any other country targeted by Big Pharma and psychiatry (an arm of industry if ever there was one) with the diligent help of the US Congress and the White House in what is a naked quid quo pro.

But the tragic fact of the matter is that this colossal, unthinkable, scam has reached the size it has, having invented diseases, gotten the public to believe in nothing else, then drugging millions upon millions of entirely normal children for behaving like children. It is an understatement, then, to say there are lots of children (and millions of adults too) who should be convinced they have been duped (all deprived of their right to informed consent) and poisoned, and that they had best get off of these poisons, and the sooner the better. Most should realize as well that they should seek to have the fraudulent diagnoses expunged from their medical records—the only true cure.

To get off of their drugs and to delete the fraudulent, stigmatizing labels, they will have to seek out physicians and mental health professionals who will outline with them a plan for weaning them from their poisons and substituting, in their place humane, human understanding, guidance and talk therapy, that credits the patient with a brain and an ability to learn, adapt and prevail. Big pharma and psychiatry have no such plan. Conveniently all of their diseases, chemical imbalances last for life and can only be controlled by chemical balancers which will be needed for life and, of course there is no talk of your learning to adapt and prevailing, emerging victorious in life.

Chapter Nine

IMMUNIZE YOUR CHILD
AGAINST ADHD

*If I could not manage a child, I thought it my ignorance
or my lack of ability as a teacher.*

- **Susan B. Anthony**

Beginning in earnest during the early 1980s, psychiatry, psychology, pediatrics, education, child protective services, and the courts have increasingly pressed the acceptance of school-based psychiatric diagnoses, and almost always for the treatment of them with powerful, dangerous drugs. For example, writing in the August 15, 2000 edition of *USA Today*, child psychiatrist Peter Jensen [1] advocates the legal enforcement of drug treatment for ADHD and other psychiatric problems diagnosed in school:

> *So what should society do if a child with a disorder with lifelong consequences is denied treatment? The answer, of course, depends on the severity of the child's condition, what other treatments have been tried and the likelihood that treatments such as Ritalin will restore that child to normal or near-normal functioning.*

The conclusion he clearly infers without stating directly is that it is okay to force drugs, whether or not the children or parents want them, so long as professionals believe the benefits outweigh the consequences. The trap here is that without a verifiable disease present the treatment becomes whatever the professionals involved say it is. And, as we have seen throughout the book, they chronically overstate the benefits of drug treatment for ADHD (there are none) and understate the risks (which are considerable). It is interesting to note that when it came to his own son, Dr. Jensen (quoted above), declined to treat him with Ritalin when the boy was diagnosed with ADHD.

What worked for ADHD is now being done for a growing number of psychiatric disorders, especially things like anxiety and bipolar. If the forcing of the ADHD diagnosis and drugs can be justified, then why not do it for every other condition? After all, it is for the good of the child, right? The problem, of course, is that with subjective diagnoses anything that disturbs adults in authority can be classified as a disease and parents threatened with the loss of their children if they don't go along with "treatment." Do any of us want this to happen, to witness childhood itself held hostage by drug pushers? We hope not.

In Aldous Huxley's *A Brave New World* citizens were issued Soma, a drug that enabled them to go through life in a state of oblivious happiness. With a potion to make them feel good all the time, there was never any reason to rebel or try to initiate any kind of change or improvements. The established order was safe. When an individual decides to live a real, Soma-free life, he is considered a criminal—just as today's drug pushing professionals seek to define any who resist the poisoning of their children.

And these drugs, be they Ritalin, Prozac, or any other on the laundry list of high profit potions, are poisons, make no mistake about it. Every drug has some degree of toxicity. For psychiatric drugs their toxic effects are unleashed on the undeveloped brains of children (but are not limited to this organ). The brain is the organ of adaptation, a wondrous, miraculous thing that changes and evolves with experience, that adjusts to its environment in order to best promote the interests of the individual in whose head it resides. To set a toxic substance loose in the brain of a child where no disease or abnormality has been found, can only impair this organ and cripple a child's efforts to adapt and succeed. It is for this reason that the psychopharmacological drugging of normal children is never justifiable. It is for this reason that no adult given true and complete disclosure of the risks and benefits of the treatment equation should ever want such drugs for themselves. It is because we invariably speak of mental/psychological symptoms in physically, medically, normal persons that the very concept of psychopharmacology is doomed never to result in net benefit, but only net harm. A brochure published by the American Academy of Neurology (of which I am a Fellow), entitled "What is a Neurologist?" reads "Protecting and treating the brain and nervous system is the essence of neurologist's work." In that the AAN is a party to psychiatry's "big lie," (having consistently refused to answer my questions, "Is ADHD a disease—yes or no?") to portray the invented disorders of the DSM to be actual diseases, leading to the drugging of millions of normal children and adults, they can hardly say they are "protecting" the brains of anyone.

Earlier in the book we saw exactly what this translated into with the Carroll family in Albany, and what the threat led to in the case of Matthew Smith's death, which opened Chapter One. A diagnosis of ADHD, or an increasing menu of other psychiatric labels, is used as justification for harassing phone calls, mistreatment of children at school, threats of state-operated children's services being unleashed, and sometimes even the loss of custody. A case could be made for this if a child had a real disease and there was a clear need for a specific treatment. But ADHD and its brethren are fictitious diseases whose diagnoses are completely subjective. This means that families face the danger of forced drugging for any child a school system has initiated the process of targeting. This means there is no abnormality for the drug to rationally, scientifically target. This means there is no science, no scientific rationale. This means the drug is a poison. What's more the leaders of psychiatry, all psychiatric researchers, and all medical scientists everywhere know of the deception and know it is poisoning. Because single mother, Diane Booth refused the ADHD-rationalized poisoning of her only child Vincent, six, Judge Leonard P. Edwards, of San Jose, made him a ward of the court and a full-time psychiatric in-patient. Nor has Diane seen him in the 5 years since. Loving, adoptive parents Linda and Robert Gale of Wilmington, North Carolina, were stripped of their adopted daughter, Angela, 12, and she, from them, over their refusal of psychiatric diagnosis and treatment. Another court-ordered kidnapping. What's more, the same thing is going on all over the country—courts kidnapping children from their parents—a payback for all of the money infusions into the government at every level from the White House and Congress down, missing not a single agent or agency. The present and past Surgeons General (the #1 federal physician) lend the weight of their position to perpetuating the disease-lie that is the linchpin of the fraud that psychiatric disorders are brain diseases, chemical imbalances, when none are—not a single one. Imagine this open-ended tool in the hands of an administration bent on subjugating all dissent. It is so much more than simply medicalizing the lives of all our normal children.

It is interesting to note that both the American Academy of Pediatrics and the American Psychological Association put their considerable weight behind legislation to make the corporal punishment of children by their parents illegal, yet have been among the featured players in the move to chemically punish children with dangerous drugs for little more than not conforming "appropriately" to the standards of adult-controlled environments. They identify normal children as having disabling, life-threatening, chemical-imbalancing, brain diseases and claim they need the equivalents of cocaine and speed to function properly. Given the physical and psychological damage this approach exposes children to, corporal punishment is much more humane in comparison.

As we have pointed out repeatedly, not a single psychiatric condition has ever been proven to be a disease. Children said to have them have never been proven to be other than normal. Calling ADHD a disease when it is not, calling children abnormal (diseased) when they are not, is a perversion of science, medicine, and morality. When normal children are drugged, whether by mistake or design, (as in the fraud of ADHD) the correct terms for what is done to them is poisoning.

For parents, being forewarned and forearmed can empower them to keep from becoming unwitting parties to the abuse of their own children. We will review what parents need to know in order to immunize their children from ADHD or, to put it more accurately, to immunize their children from those who would force dangerous drugs on them for a fraudulent diagnosis.

NOT A DISEASE — JUST A NORMAL CHILD

Diseases are natural occurrences characterized by one or more definite physical or chemical abnormalities. They result from infections, toxins, abnormal genes, cancer, or as-yet-unknown causal agents that are recognized as new diseases by astute physicians who elicit the confirmatory abnormalities upon physical examination and testing. In the case of ADHD, there is no abnormality to be found; the child is normal at the time of diagnosis, regardless of the disease lie, invariably told the parents. The first, abnormality in ADHD and in all child psychiatric "diseases"/ "chemical imbalances" comes the moment the drugs are begun—all of them powerful systemic, brain-body poisons. It is at and beyond this point that a real abnormality or abnormalities exist, depending wholly upon the number of poisons prescribed and injected or forced down the child's throat. A fake disease, then, is used as the premise for creating a real one—an intoxication, poisoning. There is never a scientific rationale for giving psychotropic drugs—never a demonstrated, diagnosed, abnormality targeted, and never a Hippocratic, moral, justification.

The promoters of ADHD like to claim they are practicing legitimate medical science because the "symptoms" of ADHD can be identified and are pronounced enough to warrant the assumption that the underlying cause will eventually be found. But this is a sham. ADHD was invented (initially as ADD) by a committee of psychiatrists and psychologists based on the belief, supported by not a speck of evidence, that normal behaviors are indicators of a neurobiological abnormality when they disturb adults. Despite regular pronouncements that its biologic roots have been discovered, no proof of a definite physical or chemical abnormality is ever offered.

All such research and all such claims, having commenced in 1970, have been a sham, meant to create illusions of science and disease while proving nothing. As we have shown in Chapter 7, the psychiatric research community, led by government researchers at the NIMH, conspired to publish studies from 1986 to the present, showing, as they knew they would, Ritalin/amphetamine-induced brain atrophy, which they, in turn, referred to as being ADHD-caused, the long-sought proof that ADHD was a brain disease.

What's more, non-psychiatrists on medical school faculties, in areas like pediatrics, internal medicine, neurology, and pathology know full well that psychiatry's claims of chemical imbalances, disorders, and diseases are a sham, their "treatment," poisoning, but say not a word. My very own alma mater, New York University has the dubious distinction of having become the preeminent ADHD center-of-excellence in the country, giving aid and comfort to disease illusionists par excellence, F. Xavier Castellanos, formerly of the NIMH, and Harold S. Koplewicz, Head of the NYU Child Study Center. But psychiatrists don't really study children. If they did, they would know and confess that there is no such thing as a psychiatric disease; what they do is drug children, one-dimensionally, for-profit.

As a parent, I challenge neurology, pediatrics, and pathology faculty members, to step forth and share an iota of proof that a single psychiatric "chemical imbalance"/ "disease" exists. Why have you and all of the rest in the medical profession stood mute as this monstrous deception, fraud, and victimization gone on? Why have you participated? There are none, at least not until their drug "treatment" commences, which is poisoning, pure and simple. What's more, all doctors, even psychiatrists, went to medical school and learned and were responsible for knowing the difference between normal and abnormal, diseased and disease-free. If they were honest with themselves, they would admit that there is no such thing as a psychiatric disease, and would stop the lying and the poisoning of normal children and normal, lied-to adults as well, and return to the tenets of their medical education and accept normal emotions, even painful ones, for what they are—the barometer of our life's-struggles for survival and happiness.

ADHD is an illusion, but if you allow yourself to be fooled into believing in it that illusion becomes a powerful force that results in very real, very serious consequences. Think about it, should your child manifest inattention, carelessness, disorganization, distractibility, fidgeting, impulsiveness, daydreaming, or anything else that makes him act any differently from a placid, yet attentive, adult, you are asked to buy into the illusion, with the process usually kicked off by a paper and pencil checklist wielded by an educator who already knows what the result will be. Mom! Dad! Think about it, is this what you want for your child?

The epidemic rages. In some classrooms 50% of the children are taking addictive drugs for ADHD, a diagnosis that did not even exist before 1980. This is the biggest health care fraud of all time, and it is being exported by US psychiatry and Big Pharma to all the rest of the world. Both the Drug Enforcement Agency and the Food and Drug Administration have acknowledged to us in writing that there is "...no proof that ADHD is a disease, a medical syndrome or anything biologic or organic." Even the ADHD "experts" (as if somebody can be an expert on something that does not exist) will not come out and say whether ADHD is a disease or not, nor will the Center for Disease Control. Yet, educators, psychologists, physicians, pharmaceutical companies, government-funded health agencies, and support groups have colluded, with the numbers of children diagnosed as ADHD increasing from 150,000 in 1970, when it was called minimal brain dysfunction, to 350,000 in 1980, the year ADD was invented, to 1 million in 1990, and, with the added impetus of ADHD in 1994, to 6 million children today. Think of it, 6 million children diagnosed with a disease in the United States, with millions more around the world, and not a single case is legitimate. Each and every diagnosis is a 100% fraud.

THE FIRST LINE OF DEFENSE: THE SCHOOLS

Your children go to school to be educated and prepared for life. It is every teacher's responsibility to discipline each child, control the class, render them literate-educable, and educate them. It is not their, or a school psychologist's, duty or within their training or capability to know beforehand who is capable of literacy and an education and who is not. Nor are they capable of knowing which children possess the capacity for self-control or do not. It is their duty to assume that all children are capable of literacy, education, and self-control and to assume responsibility, in conjunction with the parents, for helping children achieve these things. When these things are not occurring as they should, your child is in danger of receiving a diagnosis that blames all shortcomings on her or his malfunctioning brain. What a terrible thing to do to a child!

Let your child's teachers and principals know that you expect them to carry through with their responsibilities for providing an education and discipline as is age-appropriate for your child. Let them know you do not believe in, or want, any psychological/psychiatric diagnosing begun with your child, that no formal or informal mental health observations be done without your full, informed consent in advance. Tell them that if problems arise with your child to come to you with their observations and suggestions and these problems will be addressed together, in the best interest of the child, and not for the convenience of the adults who are supposed to be serving her.

BE AN ASSERTIVE PARENT/GUARDIAN

The informed consent mentioned above is an important place to assert yourself as a parent. Full, prior, informed consent means that if school personnel suggest any health or mental health evaluations or interventions they must first put their reasons in writing, along with the specifics of their recommendations. All citizens have a right to informed consent in health matters. Under this doctrine, school personnel may not begin behavioral observations for diagnostic purposes without your permission. And yet, the right of informed consent is flagrantly violated thousands of times every day. For years now schools have been practicing medicine without a license by pushing diagnoses and drugs they are not qualified to even discuss, then compound this violation by misinforming, harassing, threatening, and manipulating parents who were never consulted or given any part in the process. Why aren't parents brought in earlier? Few parents would go along with targeting their child for psychological and chemical abuse if they were fully informed.

As discussed in Chapter Three, informed consent is an essential part of your relationship with physicians and is violated at this stage, too, when doctors diagnose and prescribe without bothering to tell you that there is no evidence of ADHD's existence, while, at the same time, evidence abounds that the drugs that go with it are often addictive, always dangerous, and sometimes deadly—not the mild substances parents are led to believe they are. In any setting, the failure to provide you, the parent or guardian, with all of the material information about the "condition" or "treatment" being suggested or encouraged is a violation of your informed consent rights, which were born of the World War Two war crimes trials at Nuremberg, and is tantamount to medical malpractice. As a result of Nuremberg, medical experimentation on prisoners of war was outlawed. Today, in the 21st century, our children are not treated with this much regard, not when millions of them are functioning as subjects in a vast, for-profit medical victimization built on lies and deceit.

RATIONAL SUSPICION

With 6 million American children already diagnosed as ADHD and a few million more tagged with equally specious inventions, such as anxiety disorders and bipolar disorder, parents are not going overboard by taking proactive measures to avoid psychiatric labels and the drugs that come with them. In a 1998 article that appeared in the *Journal of the American Academy of Child and Adolescent Psychiatry* it was revealed that 97% of children who have been identified as ADHD and see a psychiatrist will be prescribed drugs—this, when non-psychiatric physicians find no evidence of physical/organic disease in a third to a half of all of their patients. This very fact shouts "beware!" Adding insult to injury, 49% end up on two or more drugs, with the additional drugs often being the off-label variety that have never been shown to be safe or effective for that age group, like the desipramine that killed Shaina Dunkle or the endless menu of substances forced on Paul Johnson, who was nearly prescribed to death.

Parents need to know that once a child has been identified the process does not end there. The special education child will have ADHD added to the mix; the ADHD child of today is the oppositional-defiant disorder young adult of tomorrow. When the ADHD drugs interfere with sleep and cause anxiety, anti-anxiety drugs and sleeping pills make up a new cocktail, and stronger stuff is yet to come if the child has more problems, maybe the heavy artillery, the anti-psychotics, will be trotted out. At no point is the only real disease addressed, encephalopathy (brain damage) resulting from the administration of Ritalin and each and every successive foreign compound without a target abnormality, the psychiatry polypharmacy for which they have been targeted from the first.

THE PREDATORS AMONG US

Not only do parents in general have to be assertive, but parents/guardians/caregivers in any situation that makes their children appear more vulnerable than average have to be especially vigilant. Remember, ADHD is a predatory phenomenon, with a gamut of adult individuals and institutions benefiting at the expense of the normal children they target, and an easy target is a more likely one.

Single and foster parents, members of minority groups, families in crisis or dysfunction, or any family perceived as relatively powerless or disenfranchised are all fair game. In these cases the harassment and threats are much more upfront, especially when additional agencies, like Child Protective Services, Social Services (and whatever equivalents exist in different states) can be called in as reinforcements when parents resist.

Do not think that just because you move out of the drug realm that the predators have been left behind. There are a growing number of "alternative" treatments that, in their own way, are equally predatory. Now, most of these approaches pose fewer physical risks than medication, which is usually their initial attraction but, just like medication, they are sold on the assumption that ADHD, or something like it, really exists and will respond to treatment.

So now chiropractors can feed at the trough, right next to the purveyors of megavitamins, special diets, biofeedback, acupuncture, and an endless list of other bogus treatments. What is called ADHD is no more due to diet, allergies, or misalignment than it is to a chemical imbalance or bad neurological wiring. Whoever tries to sell you medical, pseudo-medical, herbal, or any 'alternative' treatment for ADHD is attempting fraud, no matter if they try to con you into a drug or a diet. In all, the linchpin of the fraud is the 'Chinese menu' of brain disorders/diseases/chemical imbalances. Buy any one of them for yourself or your child and they own you, in a very real, frightening sense.

A TIGHTENING NOOSE

Here in California, Delaine Eastin, the State Superintendent of Schools threatened in 2003 to make home-schooling illegal, insisting that duly-certified teachers are essential to educate our children. Yet, hardly a day has elapsed without an article appearing to inform us that half or more of California children had performed so poorly on a high school exit exam that they were in danger of not graduating. This was hardly news in California where, in 1987, superintendent Bill Honig ordered "whole language" to the exclusion of "phonics" to teach reading and where, as evidenced on the National Assessment of Educational Progress (NAEP) throughout the nineties, California's children had become the poorest readers in the land. By the thousands and tens of thousands our children had been thwarted in their efforts to become literate and thus educable. Nor is it news when we read, year after year, that half or more of our college and community college freshmen have to take "bonehead" English (basic reading) and math to make up for teachers jobs undone in the years K-12. Nor are these the only reasons that more American families than ever before are behind the voucher movement and are "voting with their feet," enrolling their children in unprecedented numbers in private and parochial schools and home-schooling them.

The most urgent reason of all has to do with the increasingly common, coercive psychological and psychiatric diagnosing and drugging of the normal children in their trust. That they do this, instead of providing a quality education, is a total betrayal; that they do so coercively, calling in the forces of government (Child Protective Services, family and juvenile courts) and threatening law-abiding parents with loss of custody of their normal, educable children, should they resist the fraudulent labeling and drugging, is reason enough to conclude that no child and no family should be without an alternative to an United States public school education today.

The educational establishment from top to bottom should be forever ashamed of their unwitting complicity in having allowed themselves to become drug pushers in every sense of he word, in what is the greatest health care fraud in American history. Rather than gear education to the needs and aptitudes of children, they stubbornly cling to unworkable modes of education and think nothing of issuing chemical straightjackets to children who do not comply.

A WIDE RANGE OF NORMAL

If not ADHD, then what is it about so many children that results in them being identified as in the grips of a committee-created psychiatric disorder? In the overwhelming majority of cases, the underlying issue is either a clash between a normal child and the requirements of her adult-controlled environment or the product of diagnostic zeal in a newly deputized teacher-turned-deputy brain diagnostician. The sheer ecstasy of exercising such control over children and whole families is absolutely undeniable.

For parents, professionals, and even older children themselves, looking for a sound take on the issue, look no further than the wonderful *Understanding Your Child's Temperament*, by Dr. William Carey [2], Director of Behavioral Pediatrics at Children's Hospital in Philadelphia. With over 40 years experience as a pediatrician, professor, author, editor, and researcher, his approach to children is the most sensible, practical, and humane we know of. Dr. Carey has produced a considerable body of excellent work in the area of children temperaments, and tells us:

> *Temperament is the stylistic part of personality; it is the distinguishing flavor, style, or characteristic that makes one's personality unique. Temperament refers to the distinct, yet normal, behavioral patterns that we bring to various situations. It affects how we experience and respond to a multitude of environments.*

The work of Carey, and others, on temperament demonstrates that there is plenty of room for variations in behavioral styles and that what is considered normal covers a lot of territory. This is crucial because what has happened with ADHD and other psychiatric diagnoses is that the unstated definition of normal has become narrower and narrower, with the assumption made that children who fall outside of this unrealistically small territory are neurologically abnormal. The truth is that there is plenty in the normal range of temperaments that might clash with adult expectations, but that does not make it any less normal—just inconvenient for the intolerant.

Rather than tarring a child with a nonexistent brain disease and forcing her to suffer very real physical and psychological harm, we need to identify a child's unique temperament and figure out how to work with it so that her, not a teacher's or pharmaceutical company's, best interest are served. Some children have temperaments that blend well with adult-controlled institutions, which means they negotiate them without being targeted for psychiatric abuse, and some possess temperaments that clash, which has come to be the equivalent of having a bull's eye painted on one's forehead.

Because so much of temperament is inborn the amount of correcting or molding that can be done with it is limited. This doesn't mean we should forget about expecting children to follow basic norms, but it does mean their behavioral style will remain intact even after they have made whatever accommodations to adult rules they can. From here on, we need to accommodate them. Otherwise we put ourselves in opposition to what is natural to the child, which usually comes to no good. So, if a child is naturally more distractible or inattentive than others, the tendency today is to regard it as a disease to be medicated, rather than a perfectly normal variation that can be worked with.

What happens with ADHD is that the diagnostic criteria are so broad they overlap many aspects of temperament that are well within the normal range. What the ADHD criteria are measuring is not the extent of a disease or disorder, but styles of behaving that do not fit well with what adults want to see. The child who is slow to adapt to the requirements of a classroom, the child with a short attention span, he who is more active than most, she who has a more intense style of interaction, he whose moods rise and fall more frequently than average, she who happens to have greater sensitivity to others and her environment, are all in danger of being diagnosed and drugged simply for being normal when much of what is normal is no longer tolerated.

At a time when the virtues of diversity are everywhere extolled, especially in classrooms where children are lectured on how they need to embrace differences in color, ethnicity, sexual orientation, and religion, their own differences in temperament, living situations, personalities, are not tolerated at all when they clash with what adults want to see. At a time when multitudes of adults claim to be banishing bias of all kinds, a form of prejudice is being inflicted on children where they can be targeted for abuse merely for acting like normal kids.

Back in the 80s children were advised to "just say no to drugs." Early in the 21st century it is time for all of us to come together and just say no to drugging children.

Chapter Ten

I TESTIFY TO THE PARLIAMENT OF WESTERN AUSTRALIA

On June 2, 2004, I testified to Education and Health Standing Committee of the Parliament of Western Australia on the issue of ADHD diagnosis and "treatment," which is 4-5 times more common in their state than in any other state in Australia.

I began by describing the failure of both the NIMH [1] and the APA [2] to cite proof, anywhere within the scientific, medical literature that ADHD or any other psychiatric disease, is an actual disease. Then I concluded:

By now there should be no doubt that my message is simple: that no child or adult said to have a psychiatric "disorder"/ "illness"/ "syndrome"/ "disease"/ "chemical imbalance" has an abnormality/disease in a true medical sense. Instead, all of them are physically/medically normal. Further, it is this lie/perversion of science and medicine, invented and exported by US psychiatry in collusion with the pharmaceutical industry, that is the linchpin of the still-burgeoning, world-wide epidemic of psychiatric drugging/poisoning, Nor is this a matter of belief, consensus, or opinion, rather it has to do with the fact that nowhere in the scientific/medical literature of the world does replicated proof exist that ADHD or any psychiatric disorder is a physical abnormality/disease. I would add here that it is every physician's duty to prove the existence of a disease, and define that disease, before commencing with medical or surgical treatments—treatments that bear physical risks every time.

Because the burden of proof lies with those who would diagnose your children "abnormal"/ "diseased" and who would "treat" them, with addictive, dangerous, and sometimes deadly medi-

cations, and because they never provide proof, child-by-child, I would urge that you end all such "diagnosing" in your jurisdiction with the conclusions and inferences that such are physical/medical abnormalities/diseases.

DO NOT ALLOW TESTING OR LABELING: THE ONLY ABSOLUTE IMMUNITY

My message is the same to parents in the US and in every country of the world to which this fraud is being exported: do not go to those who would "screen," "examine," or "test" for their mental illnesses/disorders/diseases/chemical imbalances, for this is the process of labeling, and once labeled, the labels stick, stigmatize and enmesh you in the world of psychiatry. It all starts with the "label." That is the first "hook."

It has recently become clear that the present level of medical victimization of our own children is nowhere near sufficient for the Big Pharma-psychiatry-federal government cartel. Recall my testimony to the Health Committee of the California State Assembly of January 13, 2004: "Should you pass any law, in any way, "assuring," or sanctioning, the "diagnosis" and "treatment" of psychiatric "diseases"/ "chemical imbalances," in normal children (as is now done, California- and US-wide) or, should you fail to expunge such laws, already on the books—and you will have been a party to a fraud."

That the Congress has authored one law after another, beginning in 1970, legitimizing psychiatric disorders as diseases (and that presidents have signed them), never once requiring proof, has provided the only patina of legitimacy that such disorders/diseases have.

In Congressional hearings of May 6, 2003, William Carey, MD testified that 17 percent of US schoolchildren—9 million, were on psychiatric drugs. Not only was this not cause for revulsion in the halls of government, it was clearly an indication that their were additional millions, yet to be labeled. Just as psychiatry has sought to label and drug both parties to dysfunctional relationships, now they seek to label entire populations.

Headline: "Mentally Ill Youths 'Warehoused.'" [3] Thousands of mentally ill youths are unnecessarily put in juvenile detention centers to await mental health treatment, a House Committee reported Wednesday. "The use of juvenile detention facilities to house youth waiting for community mental health services is widespread and a serious national problem." The report was prepared at the request of California Rep. Henry Waxman, the House Government Reform Committee's top Democrat, and Sen. Susan Collins, R-Maine, chairwoman of the Senate Governmental Affairs Committee. "Thousands of youth who are in need of community mental health services are stuck in jail until these services become available," Waxman said in a statement. "This is deplorable. Congress must ensure that our children have access to the mental health care that they need."

Here the label "mentally ill" is sufficient to label and incarcerate them until mental health diagnosis and "treatment"— drugs—arrives. Just as in the foster care sector where half to two-thirds of neglected, assaulted, undereducated, entirely normal, throw-away, children are deemed mentally ill and drugged, the Big Pharma-psychiatry-government cartel has their sights on all who misbehave, keeping them imprisoned until psychiatry, bearer of labels and drugs arrives on the scene. Nor should there be any doubt that those currently without their own labels will soon get them—undoubtedly at the first psychiatric visit, just in time to make a "treatment" of the drugging to be launched with no further delay.

Let there be no doubt; every agent and agency of the federal government is involved. President Bush, convinced that the drugging of 17% of the nations 52 million schoolchildren is too many children "left behind"(giving new meaning to "no child left behind") has just launched his own plan to screen all children and employees in the nation's public schools for mental illness: "Bush plans to screen whole US population for mental illness." [4]

As if we spoke of actual diseases, President Bush's New Freedom Commission on Mental Health, has just announced that "despite their prevalence, mental disorders often go undiagnosed" and recommends comprehensive mental health screening for "consumers of all ages," including preschool children. "Each year," they say, "young children are expelled from preschools and childcare facilities for severely disruptive behaviors and emotional disorders." These are the ones, we have no doubt, being held in prisons until psychiatric "diagnosis" and "treatment" can arrive—but hopefully not those expelled from preschools. The commission also recommended "linkage [of screening] with "treatment and supports" including "state-of-the-art treatments" using "specific medications for specific conditions."

The problem is there is nothing specific about psychiatric conditions. None of them are actual diseases. And yet, for 35 years, from 1970 to the present, Congress has enacted (and past presidents have signed) laws assuring the diagnosis and drug treatment of psychiatric disorders, alleged to be diseases, while never once requiring proof that they are. Thus it is that the millions of children said to have ADHD and all psychiatric disorders, are physically, medically, normal until such time as their "treatment"/drugging commences. In other words, the lives of millions upon millions of normal children, in the US and around the world, are needlessly, destructively, medicalized in the name of psychiatric diagnosis and treatment.

Clearly, there is a need to immunize all normal children everywhere. Nor is this a scientific debate—there is no science. Nor is it a matter of misstating the safety and efficacy of medications; with no diseases to target they are not "medications" they are foreign compounds—poisons, each with its greater or lesser potential to harm or kill.

Recall the words of Dr. John D. Griffith Assistant Professor of Psychiatry, Vanderbilt University School of Medicine: "I would like to point out that every drug, however innocuous, has some degree of toxicity. A drug, therefore, is a type of poison and its poisonous qualities must be carefully weighed against its therapeutic usefulness." This is just as is known by all professors of medicine and pharmacology, just as is known by all who have graduated from medical school.

Once again, and this cannot be stated too often, the linchpin of the fraud, the "big lie," is calling all things—emotional, behavioral, mental, psychological, psychiatric—brain abnormalities/diseases/chemical imbalances, when none are, not a single one. The only reason I can see that psychiatrists go to medical school, is to learn to speak medical-ese, so as to carry out the "disease" lie.

It is this lie which, in and of itself, defeats informed consent and make the deceived patient/parents an involuntary conscript in psychiatric-pharmaceutical bondage, to some extent, permanently, in every single case. The sheer numbers of such victims in this modern-day horror story are unbelievable, as is the extent of their reach, which is without limit. Having appended one label and prescribed one drug for all 52 million in US public schools, I have no doubt that they would call this under-diagnosis and under-treatment and set about to screen them again so as not to miss the 2nd and 3rd, co-morbid (co-existent) disorders/diseases/chemical imbalances, so as to have semantic justification—if nothing else—for the 2nd, 3rd, and 5th chemical balancers they have in their armamentarium.

Recalling that invariable psychological harm is done by the label itself which asks that the child, their parents, family, school and community believe there is something abnormal/diseased about their brain that renders it impossible for them control themselves without a chemical balancer—pill—or 2 or 3 or 5 or 6.

They can never justify medicating (actually poisoning) without a medical diagnosis—an abnormality/disease/chemical imbalance. And for this reason they cannot confess to having no disease on the risk side of the risk vs. benefit equation and justify prescribing a medication with all of the risks listed in the *Physician's Desk Reference*. After all, every drug in the **PDR** has known side effects and contraindications running to 1-4 fine-print lines, 11 inches tall. And these mind you are just the side effects they admit to. Were they to add the dangers spoken of from their post-marketing experience, such as the 186 deaths due to methylphenidate (Ritalin) during the decade 1990-2000, how many drugs would they sell? Very few, I assure you.

This is why they must be cut off at the pass—don't go for the mental illness screening! Send a letter to school the day your child starts, saying under no circumstances is my child to be evaluated, no matter how formally or informally, for any mental illness or any mental health purpose. Make clear in your letter that you—the parents will make all decisions regarding your child's health care needs, physical and otherwise, and that you will not be delegating such decision making to any other party, least of all school personnel—teachers, therapists, and psychologists.

The aim here is to prevent "labeling" from ever taking place, for once it has, the wheels are in motion for them to push for "treatment," a push so strong, few parents and families, can truly resist it, and mind you, as in the cases of the Carroll family, Diane and Vincent Booth, and Gail and Robert Suarez, they have the local court, Child Protective Services and law enforcement on their side, and once in that venue, the chance that you can actually win, retaining control of the life of your child, is virtually zero. This is why the only way to provide your child/children with full immunity is to prevent all mental health labeling!

I have a good friend Hideo Sasahara, from Japan, whose son, now in his early twenties was labeled ADHD, but never drugged. Nonetheless the label has stuck, indelibly in his son's record, causing many, such as potential employers, and sellers of health and other insurance to view him, in real-world terms as somehow brain-impaired. Even with the expensive help of attorneys, he is finding it impossible to remove the fraudulent, ADHD label.

I have no doubt that had Kelly and Larry Smith been told, honestly and factually, that their son Matthew was normal, and that ADHD was nothing but a set of bothersome behaviors, that they would never have allowed the poisoning of their son, and he would be alive today.

Had Janet and Michael Hall been told the truth about Stephanie—that she was normal, that there was no such thing as ADHD–a disease, that they would never have allowed her poisoning with Ritalin, and she would have lived to see her 11th birthday and a lifetime of birthdays.

I have no doubt that had Vicky and Steve Dunkle been told that their daughter, Shaina was normal—that she had no disease—that one look at the PDR litany of side effects regarding desipramine, that they would never have allowed a single such pill to cross her lips, and she too would be alive today.

Jackie Morgan was led to believe ADHD was a disease. She was duped—yes—by physicians she should have been able to trust. Had she not, she wouldn't have allowed the desipramine poisoning of her son, Cameron Pettus, and he too would be alive today. This is all it would have taken. No mention of the growing numbers of normal children dying, suddenly, of heart attacks would have been needed; no mention of the debate within psychiatry to ban this poison would have been needed; Cameron would be alive today.

What's more, Randy Steel, Eric Martin, Shannon Sizemore, Travis Neal, Macauley Showalter, and all of the countless thousands killed this way, would still be alive and normal, just as they were when ADHD was diagnosed, before the Ritalin/amphetamine poisoning. Had all of their parents been told the truth—that ADHD (and every other psychiatric "disorder") was not a disease, had never been a disease, would never be a disease—the truth they needed to make an informed decision, the truth they deserved, but did not get, they would all be alive and healthy today.

I often think how lucky I (FB) was to have gone to public school before the days of its takeover by psychology and psychiatry. To be sure, I and others acted up at times, and the situations needed understanding and were understood by our teachers, and we were dealt with accordingly, without psychology, psychiatry or the drugs. What's more, we learned to read and to do math and if we didn't, our teachers and parents knew the reasons why. What's more no epidemics of ADHD-afflicted, dyslexia-afflicted, dycalculia-afflicted, CD-, ODD-, bipolar-, clinical depression-, or OCD-afflicted children were graduated into the ranks of the high schools we went on to. We had mental health in spades, far more than all of the psychologists and psychiatrists I have known since.

It should be apparent that we must, at all costs, not allow them to label any child with their anti-scientific, anti-human being, anti-civil rights labels. Here is where they must be stopped. Furthermore, with Congress and the President fomenting the fraudulent labeling, we must stand together, to stop this assault on American life that is so far along as to be nearly unbelievable.

Chapter Eleven

ALERT! ADDERALL CAUSES 20 DEATHS AND 12 STROKES!

On February 9, 2005, Health Canada, the Canadian counterpart of the FDA, instructed Britain's Shire Pharmaceuticals Group Plc, manufacturer of Adderall and Adderall–XR (both a mixture of amphetamine salts), to withdraw Adderall–XR (the long-acting form—the only one sold in Canada) from the Canadian market. Their decision came after a review of 20 sudden deaths (14 in children) and 12 strokes (2 in children) in patients taking either Adderall or Adderall–XR. Nor were these occurrences associated with overdose, misuse or abuse—they were being taken as directed.

What of US children—should they be taking it?

Dr. Robert Temple of the FDA in the February 14, 2005, *Los Angeles Times* stated the FDA is aware that children have died after taking the drug, but cannot tell whether the rate is higher than it is in the general population. "There is a background rate of sudden death in children," he explained.

The *Fresno Bee* (February 11, 2005) reported: "Officials at the Food and Drug Administration asked Canadian regulators to refrain from suspending the use of the hyperactivity drug Adderall XR, because the FDA could not handle another 'drug safety crisis.'" Meanwhile, the FDA is allowing the drug's sales to continue in the United States. A million children in the US are taking one form or the other of Adderall, almost always for ADHD.

An FDA web site advisory explains: "Of 12 total cases, five occurred in patients with underlying structural heart defects (abnormal arteries or valves, abnormally thickened walls, etc.), all conditions that increase the risk for sudden death. Several of the remaining cases presented problems of interpretation, including a family history of ventricular tachycardia (rapid heart rate), association of death with heat exhaustion, dehydration and near-drowning, very rigorous exercise, fatty liver, heart attack, and type 1 diabetes mellitus. One case was reported three to four years after the event and another had above-toxic blood levels of amphetamine. The duration of treatment varied from one day to 8 years. The number of cases of sudden deaths reported for Adderall is only slightly greater, per million prescriptions, than the number reported for methylphenidate (Ritalin, Concerta, Metadate) products, which are also commonly used to treat pediatric patients with ADHD."

This sounds as if the FDA is bending over backwards to exonerate Adderall.

Over the same time period, 1999-2003, the FDA's reporting system recorded seven sudden deaths of children taking other ADHD stimulants—Concerta, sold by Johnson & Johnson and Ritalin, made by Novartis AG. All three drugs are Schedule II psychostimulants, and all are known to be highly addictive, dangerous and deadly. The FDA MedWatch program, one of voluntary physician reporting, is judged to detect no more than one to ten percent of side effects of a given drug. There were 186 deaths related to methylphenidate/Ritalin between 1990 and 2000.

Psychologist William Pelham of the University at Buffalo urged that parents take a hard look at whether their children really need these medications. He points out that behavioral training programs for children, parents and teachers can lessen the need for drugs or make them unnecessary [www.wings.buffalo.edu/adhd]. Suggesting that behavioral training might render drugs unnecessary is to suggest that ADHD is a behavioral problem, not a physical-medical abnormality, a disease which, of course, is the fact of the matter.

As news of deaths—this time from Adderall—emerge, it is time to demand that the FDA, NIMH, and NIH, confess to the public that ADHD is not and never has been a disease. This means, of course, that virtually none of the drugs said to be "essential" treatment for ADHD have a positive "risk" vs. "benefit" ratio needed to justify their use. All of the Schedule II, amphetamine and amphetamine-like drugs are highly addictive, damage both brain and body and cause death—mostly cardiovascular deaths. Given that ADHD "patients" are medically, physically normal, these drugs are actually not justifiable. Even the supposed "non-stimulant" Strattera has recently been found to be liver-toxic, its use not justifiable in normals.

That the FDA is a party to the fraud of calling psychiatric diagnoses, diseases, is seen in the informed consent document already in use for the recently launched FDA-approved study: "Effect of Single Dose of Dextroamphetamine in Attention Deficit Hyperactivity Disorder: a functional magnetic resonance study" (NIH study 2514-1 (4-97) PA 09-25-0099), which reads: "Your child is invited to volunteer in an outpatient research study examining the effects of a single dose of dextroamphetamine on brain activation patterns in healthy children and children with ADHD." Saying, "in healthy children and children with ADHD" they infer that those with ADHD are other than healthy, i.e., diseased, abnormal. Saying, "Dextroamphetamine is a psycho-stimulant that has been approved by the FDA for the treatment of ADHD in both children and adolescents," they infer ADHD is something that needs treatment, i.e., a disease/abnormality. Saying, "Your child has been asked to participate because he/she has been diagnosed with ADHD," they infer that having ADHD is to have a disease/abnormality. Saying, "The purpose of this study is to compare brain activity between healthy children and children with ADHD," they infer that children with ADHD are unhealthy/diseased and that their brain activity (as seen on f-MRI scanning) is abnormal. Saying "Compare the effects of a single dose of dextroamphetamine on brain activity in healthy children and children with ADHD" they once again infer children with ADHD are unhealthy, diseased. Saying, "Examine whether the differences in brain activity between children with ADHD and healthy children are caused by the symptoms of ADHD or by genes that affect brain activity," they leave no doubt ADHD is viewed as an abnormality/disease, one due to a defective gene or genes, affecting the electrical activity of the brain. Leading subjects in a study to believe they have an organic disease when what they have are symptoms that are psychogenic or situationally caused, invalidates their informed consent, biases them in favor of biological treatments, and against psychological/behavioral treatments and, irrefutably, invalidates the study itself, which should lead to cessation of the study.

On December 24, 1994, Paul Leber, of the FDA wrote me: "...as yet no distinctive pathophysiology for the disorder has been delineated."

Recall from Chapter 7, "The Final Statement of the NIH, ADHD, Consensus Conference Panel, November 18, 1998," which read: ...we do not have an independent, valid test for ADHD, and there are no data to indicate that ADHD is due to a brain malfunction. Nor has there been validation of ADHD as a disease since—proof, repeatedly, that amphetamines and methylphenidate cause grossly evident brain atrophy—"Yes!" but never, confirmation of psychiatry's and the pharmaceutical industry's wishful thinking that ADHD is a bona fide disease.

AMPHETAMINES AND THE HEART

The FDA advisory on Adderall continues: "... the FDA has not decided to take any further regulatory action at this time. However, because it appeared that patients with underlying heart defects might be at increased risk for sudden death, the labeling for Adderall XR was changed in August, 2004 to include a warning that these patients might be at particular risk, and that these patients should ordinarily not be treated with Adderall products." Saying underlying heart defects they assume and lead the public to believe that the heart defects of which they speak were present before treatment with Adderall was begun. They must state—but have not—what, exactly these heart defects were, and whether they were diagnosed (1) during life, prior to all drug treatment, (2) during life, after treatment with Adderall or any drugs, was begun, or, (3) at autopsy, leaving the distinct possibility that the "underlying heart defects" mentioned, might also have been caused by the Adderall (amphetamine) exposure.

In *The Pathology of Drug Abuse*, Karch writes: "Amphetamine's adverse effects on the heart are well established ...(sharing) common mechanisms with cocaine toxicity...cardiomyopathy seems to be a complication of amphetamine abuse more often than cocaine abuse...The clinical history in most of these cases is consistent with arrhythmic sudden death [as in the case of Stephanie Hall]. Reports of amphetamine-related sudden death were first published shortly after amphetamine became commercially available" [in the late 1930s, about the same time Bradley discovered the paradoxical, calming effect of amphetamines that has lead to today's Ritalin epidemic]....Stimulant-related cardiomyopathy has occurred in association with amphetamine, methamphetamine...and methylphenidate [see case of 13 year-old Matthew Smith, coerced by educators to stay on Ritalin]...In all cases there was acute onset of heart failure associated with decreased cardiac output..."

Of 2,993 adverse reaction (AR) reports concerning "Ritalin" or "methylpenidate" listed by the FDA's Division of Pharmacovigilance and Epidemiology (DPE), from 1990 to 1997, there were 160 deaths and 569 hospitalizations—36 of them life-threatening. One hundred twenty-six (126) were cardiovascular occurrences, and 949 central or peripheral nervous system occurrences. There were 6 cases of "cardiomyopathy," 12 of "arrhythmia," 7 of "bradycardia" (slow pulse), 5 of "bundle branch block" (impairment of conduction apparatus of the heart), 4 of "EKG abnormality,"

5 "extrasystole" (heart rhythm abnormalities), 3 "heart arrest," 2 heart failure, right," 10 "hypotension" (low BP), 1 "myocardial infarction," 15 "tachycardia" (rapid pulse).

Other such molecules include fenfluramine (Pondimin)—the 'fen' of 'fen-phen'—the weight reduction compound found to cause heart valve defects, leading to its being withdrawn from the market. There have been reports of reversible cardiomyopathy with methamphetamine (Desoxyn, Gradumet); of cardiomyopathy with dextro-amphetamine (Dexedrine) or, of left ventricular failure following a single, i.v. dose of amphetamine.

Are these—Adderall-caused, amphetamine-caused, cardiovascular abnormalities, the "underlying heart defects" the FDA has cautioned, must never be "treated" with Adderall? Clearly, the FDA owes all available facts about these supposedly preexisting, supposedly "underlying heart defects," to the US public.

NEVER EVER DUE TO ADHD OR ANY PSYCHIATRIC "DISEASE"/ "CHEMICAL IMBALANCE"

As powerful and long-lived as the psychiatric "disease"/ "chemical imbalance" lie has been, we must debunk it. Not a single such entity in any edition of the DSM is an actual disease/ biological, physical, organic, abnormality and, for that reason none, in and of themselves, can be the cause of a heart defect or of any physical defect found at any time in the life (or at autopsy) of a psychiatric patient. All such abnormalities/diseases must either be an independent, coincidental disease (such as cancer, multiple sclerosis, or asbestosis), or due to a psychiatric drug or drugs they have been on. The litany of side-effects for every drug in the *Physician's Desk Reference* are always a result of the drug exposure, never of the psychiatric "disease" itself, for the simple reason, that none are actual diseases. It is this fraud, among others, that the FDA has been an eager party to.

FDA—PARTNER IN
VICTIMIZATION OF THE PUBLIC

In the late fifties thalidomide became the sleeping pill of choice, primarily in the UK and continental Europe, but actually worldwide. Soon there followed an epidemic of thousands of newborns with phocomelia—seal-like congenital amputations, previously almost unheard of. After rounds of denials from the drug's various manufacturers, the persistence of Professor Widikund Lenz, a German geneticist, made clear the causal association of the drug. Only then, in 1960, was thalidomide banned around the world. There were up to 12,000 cases worldwide. But the US was spared. Reviewing the world's literature on thalidomide, Dr. Frances Kelsey of the FDA found reason for alarm and lead the FDA refusal to license thalidomide for marketing in the US. But we saw occasional cases in the US, largely in the offspring of Armed Forces families stationed abroad; and there were cases aplenty in Canada, many of which were seen in amputee clinics in the states. That was the late fifties and early sixties. The FDA no doubt protected the public good. The drug companies urging FDA approval and marketing did not win out.

What about today? I doubt the FDA would have banned thalidomide. Just as they do today with addictive, dangerous, and deadly, but non-essential, drugs (sleeping pills, pain pills, psychiatric pills), they would have found a way to champion the marketplace cause of thalidomide.

In the mid-nineties they resisted calls to ban the pediatric use of tricyclic antidepressants despite reports of sudden deaths, such as in the cases of Shaina Dunkle and Cameron Pettus.

In 1998, the FDA was forced to remove three drugs from the market because of safety problems, more than in any similar period in its history. Redux for causing heart valve defects, Posicor for causing life-threatening drug interactions and fatal heart problems, and Duract, for causing sometimes-fatal liver damage. None represented a significant advance in effectiveness, and in all three cases, significant safety concerns existed prior to approval. Congress, another protector of the pharmaceutical industry, more so than of the public, has systematically weakened a drug-approval process that for years ensured Americans the safest pharmaceutical supply in the world. When Rezulin, one of 11 drugs available to treat diabetes, caused 33 deaths due to liver failure, Britain, but not the US, had the good sense to ban it.

All ADHD drugs now in use in the US have serious side effects not appropriately addressed by the FDA.

Cylert (pemoline), found to cause liver failure and death was banned in Canada, but not the US. Strattera, a non-stimulant addition to the ADHD armamentarium was touted as non-addictive and safe until it was discovered in recent months, after being marketed, to cause liver toxicity.

The SSRI antidepressants, Celexa, Lexapro, Paxil and Zoloft, found by British authorities to be of little or no effectiveness and to increase the rate of suicide have all been banned with the exception of Prozac for childhood use. Predictably, the FDA, holding, as does Surgeon General Richard Carmona, that "childhood depression" is an actual brain disease, has taken no such action.

I have come to the conclusion that the US public would be better off without the FDA. But this will not happen for they are an essential, for-profit tool to its collaborators—government and the pharmaceutical industry—to, author and defend the illusion of drug efficacy and safety, no matter how dangerous and deadly, as long as the bottom line is healthy. This, literally and figuratively, is a sickening state of affairs, one I never imagined I would see when I graduated medical school and entered the medical profession in 1960.

THE ADHD FRAUD
ENDNOTES & REFERENCES

Chapter 1

1. "Amphetamine's adverse effects on the heart are well established...(sharing) common mechanisms with cocaine toxicity...cardiomyopathy seems to be a complication of amphetamine abuse more often than cocaine abuse...The clinical history in most of these cases is consistent with arrhythmic sudden death (see case of Stephanie Hall). Reports of amphetamine-related sudden death were first published shortly after amphetamine became commercially available" (late 1930s, about the same time Bradley discovered the paradoxical, calming effect of amphetamines that has lead to today's Ritalin epidemic)...Stimulant-related cardiomyopathy has occurred in association with amphetamine, methamphetamine...and methylphenidate (Ritalin)...In all cases there was acute onset of heart failure associated with decreased cardiac output." See Karch, SB. *The Pathology of Drug Abuse*, 2nd ed. (CRC Press, 1996), p. 2.

2. Ritalin and other amphetamines can interfere with the body phospholipid chemistry causing the accumulation of abnormal membranes visible with an electron microscope. Such abnormalities were seen in an adult treated with Ritalin for 4 ½ years in whom a heart muscle biopsy was obtained during coronary bypass surgery. Fischer concluded: "... we feel the methylphenindate (Ritalin) should be considered as the incriminating factor since this agent is amphetamine-related." See Fischer, VW, et al., "Cardiomyopathic Findings Associated With Methylpheni-

date," *Journal of the American Medical Association* 238
(1977):1497). Henderson et al., next exposed experimental
mice and rats to methylphenidate (Ritalin), and found
identical membrane proliferation to that in the patient
described by Fischer (1977). Moreover, they found that
"The methylphenidate (Ritalin) doses used in the experimental rodents fell within the range of therapeutic dosage prescribed for patients with attention deficit disorders
(ADD/ADHD)." See Henderson, TA, et. al., "Effects of
Methylphenidate on Mammalian Myocardial Ultrastruc-
ture," *The American Journal of Cardiovascular Pathology*
5 (1994): 68-78.

3. "Whereas the majority of children experience only minor side
effects under medically supervised controlled conditions,
there are a significant number of case reports document-
ing more severe abuse. These reports and scientific studies
of abuse potential are routinely down-played, if referenced
at all. As a consequence, parents of children and adult
patients are not being provided with the opportunity for
informed consent or a true risk/benefit consideration in
deciding whether methylphenidate (or any amphetamine)
therapy is appropriate." See *DEA Background Paper on
Methylphenidate*, Drug Enforcement Administration, US
Department of Justice, Drug and Chemical Evaluation
Section, Office of Diversion Control, p 8.

4. "Psychostimulant therapy did not significantly improve the
outcome measures (GPAs) in the cohort diagnosed with
predominantly inattentive ADHD and academic impairment. Additional comorbidities were diagnosed and treated,
but differences among participants were not statistically
significant. Short-term decreases in DSM-IV symptoms of
predominantly inattentive ADHD did not translate into
academic gains." See McCormick, LH. "ADHD treatment

and academic performance: a case series," *Journal of Family Practice* 52 (August, 2003): 620-24, 626. Although short-duration methylphenidate and amphetamine studies have shown educational improvement, this has not been true of studies lasting longer than three months. See McBride, et al. "Serotonergic responsivity in male young patients with autistic behavior," *Archives of General Psychiatry* 46 (1989): 213-21. Multi-year studies have failed to show persistent benefits in academic or social areas for children who stay on stimulant therapy. Such studies have been limited due to their retrospective nature and failure to monitor compliance with pill-taking. See Schachar, R and Tannock, R. "Childhood hyperactivity and psychostimulants: a review of extended treatment studies," *Journal of Child and Adolescent Psychopharmacology* 3 (1993): 81-97. Likewise, Carlson and Bunner acknowledge short-term, but not long-term, academic gains. See Carlson, CL and Bunner, M. "Effects of methylphenidate on the academic performance of children with attention-deficit hyperactivity disorder," *School Psychology Review* 22 (1993): 184-98. Educational enhancement cannot be given as a reason for stimulant or any psychotropic drug treatment.

5. It is commonly assumed that a child's response to Ritalin/amphetamine treatment confirms a diagnosis of ADHD. This was disproved in 1978 when it was shown that normal children's responses to stimulants are identical to those of children with ADHD. As we now know, there is no physical difference between normals and children said to have ADHD. See Rapoport, JL, et al. "Dextroamphetamine: cognitive and behavioral effects in normal prepubertal boys," *Science* 199 (1978): 560-63 and Zametkin, AJ. "Attention-Deficit Disorder: Born to Be Hyperactive?," *JAMA* 273 (June 21, 1995): 1871-74.

6. Ingestion of androstenedione can increase the levels of male and female sex hormones. Athletes take the supplement for muscle building. Potential long-term consequences of androstenedione use in men include testicular atrophy, impotence, and feminization. Women can experience masculinization and also are at risk for menstrual abnormalities, blood clots, and breast and endometrial cancer. In a 2002 survey conducted by the National Institute on Drug Abuse, approximately one in 40 high school seniors acknowledged having used androstenedione during the past year. See "FDA Is Cracking Down on Manufacturers of "Andro," *Clinical Psychiatric News* (June, 2004): 81. In "performance enhancement," just as in psychiatry, the only abnormality/disease is that caused by the drugs.

7. *MedWatch.* The Food and Drug Administration Medical Products Reporting Program, Division of Pharmacovigilance and Epidemiology (DPE) 1990-1997; 1998-2000.

8. As the main speaker at the November 16-18, 1998, NIH Consensus Conference on ADHD, on the subject "Is ADHD a Valid Disorder?," William B. Carey concluded: "...common assumptions about ADHD include that it is clearly distinguishable from normal behavior, constitutes a neuro-developmental disability, is relatively uninfluenced by the environment—all of these assumptions...must be challenged because of the weakness of empirical (research) support and the strength of contrary evidence...What is now most often described as ADHD in the United States appears to be a set of normal behavioral variations... This discrepancy leaves the validity of the construct (ADHD) in doubt..."

9. "Who else exercises such vast discretionary powers over his fellow man as the contemporary psychiatrist?" See Szasz, Thomas. *The Manufacture of Madness—A Comparative Study of the Inquisition and the Mental Health Movement* (Harper and Row, 1970), p. 62. Today, teachers, all of them "deputy diagnosticians," are likewise drunk with power as they routinely mandate and coerce life-changing diagnoses and treatments.

10. The percent of children with proneness to crying increased by ten percent during a course of low-dose methylphenidate (Ritalin) treatment. See Barkley, RA, et al. "Side effects of methylphenidate with attention deficit disorder: a systematic, placebo-controlled evaluation," *Pediatrics* 86 (1990):184-92. In a partially controlled study, 18.8% were lethargic, 26.1 % were irritable, and 7.0% had severe reactions. See Mayes, SD, et al. "Methylphenidate and ADHD: influence of age, IQ and neurodevelopmental status," *Developmental Medicine and Child Neurology* 36 (1994):1099-1107. Ten percent of study participants dropped out. See Schachar, RJ, et al. "Behavioral, situational, and temporal effects of treatment of ADHD with methylphenidate," *Journal of the American Academy of Child and Adolescent Psychiatry* 36 (1997): 754-63. 4.8% developed hallucinations. See Gillberg, C, et al. "Long-term stimulant treatment of children with attention-deficit hyperactivity disorder symptoms: a randomized, double-blind, placebo-controlled trial," *Archives of General Psychiatry* 54 (1997): 857-64. In another study, 6 of 98 children on stimulant therapy, for an average of 21 months, developed psychotic symptoms. In none could the psychotic symptoms have been due to ADHD for the simple reason that ADHD has never been proved to be a disease. See Cherland, E and Fitzpatrick, R. "Psychotic Side Effects of

Psychostimulants: A 5-Year Review," *Canadian Journal of Psychiatry* 44 (1999): 811–13.

11. The combination of clonidine (Catapres) with methylphenidate was scrutinized following the report of 3 deaths in children whose treatment included this combination. See Swanson, JM, et al. "Clonidine in the Treatment of ADHD: Questions about Safety and Efficacy" [letter to the editor], *Journal of Child and Adolescent Psychopharmacology* 5 (1995):301-4 and Swanson, Jm, et al."Combining Methylphenidate and Clonidine: Ill-Advised," *Journal of theAmerican Academy of Child and Adolescent Psychiatry* 38 (1999): 617.

12. Having been on Ritalin for 7 years Rod Matthews wrote to his teacher: "I like to do crazy things, I've been lighting fires, I've been wanting to kill people I hate." Rod's story went on to state, "Thoughts of suicide troubled him, something he never experienced before taking the drug. He finally selected a target — a new boy in the neighborhood, Shaun Ouillette. Yet, the warning signs — like the ominous letter in teacher Triconi's box — escaped unnoticed. Then, on November 20, 1986, Rod lured Shaun into a forested area. Rod followed in the footsteps of the larger boy. Deep in the woods— far from any possible help for his victim — Rod swung his bat. Shaun fell to his knees, crying "God help me!" Again and again Rod smashed him, leaving the body where it fell. Tried as an adult and convicted of second-degree murder, Rod became the youngest inmate in the Massachusetts prison system, refused parole, time and again. Rod Matthews "was a nice, good kid. There was nothing angry or violent or aggressive about him until the ADHD diagnosis and the Ritalin prescription that went with it." See Whittle,

Thomas and Amato, Linda. "Education: The Fatal Flaw," *Freedom Magazine* 36 (number 1): 7-15.
Ten days after he began taking Adderall to control his attention deficit Ryan Ehlis slipped into a psychotic fog and killed his infant daughter. He was then acquitted of murder by a judge who ruled his psychotic state was a rare side effect of Adderall. See Witte, Brian. "Slaying Blamed on Drug Reaction." Bismarck, North Dakota, *AP News Service* (October 26, 1999). These are dangerous, deadly drugs we feed, so casually, and without the least medical justification, to millions of our very own, entirely normal, children. Not only is informed consent a right it is a duty, when, as parents, we are the primary protectors of our children.

13. Stubbe DE, Thomas WJ. "A Survey of Early-career Child and Adolescent Psychiatrists: Professional Activities and Perceptions." *Journal of the American Academy of Child and Adolescent Psychiatry* 2002 Feb;41(2):123-30.

Chapter 2

1. "Nevertheless, all across America we have the spectacle of an entire generation of little boys, by the tens of thousands, being dosed up on ADD's magic bullet of choice, Ritalin, the CIBA-Geneva Corporation's brand name for the stimulant methylphenidate. I first encountered Ritalin in 1966 when I was in San Francisco doing research for a book on the psychedelic or hippie movement. A certain species of the genus hippie was known as the Speed Freak, and a certain strain of Speed Freak was known as the Ritalin Head. The Ritalin Heads loved Ritalin. You'd see them in the throes of absolute Ritalin raptures...Not a wiggle, not a peep...They would sit engrossed in anything at all...a manhole cover, their own

palm wrinkles...indefinitely...through shoulda-been meal-time after mealtime...through raging insomnias...Pure methylphenidate nirvana..." See Wolfe, Tom. *Hooking Up*. (Farrar Strauss & Giroux), 2000.

2. Child psychiatrist, Peter S. Jensen, advocates the legal enforcement of drug treatment for ADHD and other psychiatric problems diagnosed in school. He writes: "So what should society do if a child with a disorder with lifelong consequences is denied treatment?" Here, is Jensen implying that ADHD is a "disorder" by which he means "disease," having "lifelong consequences" demanding "treatment?" "Opposing View" 2000, (August 15), *USA Today*, 16A.

3. The majority children who take Ritalin or an amphetamine become subdued, over-focused, and compliant—no longer child-like, which means they are no longer normal, but have drug-induced, abnormal behavior due to a diffuse, drug-induced, organic, abnormality of the brain.

4. See Carey, WB. "Is ADHD a Valid Disorder?" *National Institute of Health (NIH), Consensus Conference on ADHD* (November 16-18, 1998).

5. See "Sudden death in children treated with a tricyclic antidepressant," *The Medical Letter on Drugs and Therapeutics* 32 (815), (1990): 53.

6. See Riddle, MA, et al. "Sudden death in children receiving Norpramin: a review of three reported cases and commentary," *Journal of the American Academy of Child and Adolescent Psychiatry* 30 (1990): 104-8.

7. See Werry, JS, et al., "Resolved cardiac arrhythmias make desipramine an unacceptable choice in children, "*Journal*

of the American Academy of Child and Adolescent Psychiatry 34 (1995): 1245-48.

8. See Wilens, TE, et al. "Combined pharmacotherapy: an emerging trend in pediatric psychopharmacology," *Journal of the American Academy of Child and Adolescent Psychiatry* 34 (1995): 110-12.

Chapter 3

1. See *Federal Involvement in the Use of Behavior Modification Drugs on Grammar School Children of The Right to Privacy Inquiry Hearing Before Subcommittee on The Committee on Government Operations* House of Representatives, 91st Congress, Second Session September 29, 1970.

2. Healy, David. *The Creation of Psychopharmacology.* (Harvard University Press, 2002).

3. *Diagnostic and Statistical Manual of Mental Disorders*, 3rd Edition, (American Psychiatric Association, 1980)

4. Carey, William and McDevitt, Sean. *Coping with Children's Temperament* (Basic Books, 1995).

5. On April 28, 1992, Congresswoman Patricia Schroeder, D-Colorado, chaired hearings before the Select Committee on Children, Youth, and Families, the proceedings subsequently published under the title: *The Profits of Misery: How Inpatient Psychiatric Treatment Bilks the System and Betrays our Trust.* Dr. Walter E. Afield, psychiatrist, chief executive officer, and medical director of the Mental Health Program Corporation of Tampa, Florida, testified: "However, there are abuses going on nationwide in our mental health system that are terrible, whether you're talking about equestrian therapy or you're talking about sex addiction in a hospital in New Orleans. That's not

even in the DSM III. The DSM III, we're talking about everyone in this room will fit into two or three of the diagnoses in the DSM III. That's what's so vague about the situation, and it changes. In DSM II, homosexuality was a disease. In III, it's not. In [DSM] IV there'll be some new diseases. Every new disease that's defined gets a new hospital program, new admissions and a new system and a way to bilk it, and this bilking continues and it's a combination of who owns these places and it's also a combination of the way the doctors are trained."

6. See "Basic Nomenclature Issues of the DSM IV: How to define "mental disorder," *Clinical Psychiatric News* (August 2002): 5 "The DSM has never contained a detailed definition that is useful as a criterion for deciding what is, or is not, a mental disorder." This shocking confession can be taken as having come directly from the DSM Committee of the American Psychiatric Association.

7. See *Federal Involvement in the Use of Behavior Modification Drugs on Grammar School Children of The Right to Privacy Inquiry Hearing Before Subcommittee on The Committee on Government Operations*, House of Representatives 91st Congress, Second Session September 29, 1970 (chaired by Rep. Cornelius Gallagher).

8. See Cowell, Alan. "House of Lords puts limits, not ban, on parents hitting kids," *New York Times News Service*, July 6, 2004. There can be no doubt that biologically-bent psychology and psychiatry have been behind attempts to criminalize and ban corporal punishment, even by parents of their own children, so as to make way for their drugging enterprise.

9. Here we see the diagnosis of a psychiatric "diseases" as the linchpin of the fraud. Each is justification for prescription

medication. Even in the rare instances in which teachers don't frankly mention a "disease" or drug, they urge that the child be seen by a physician—usually one known to the school as an ADHD/mental health expert.

10. *Diagnostic and Statistical Manual of Mental Disorders*, 3rd edition-revised (DSM-III-R). (American Psychiatric Association), 1987.

11. *Diagnostic and Statistical Manual of Mental Disorders*, 4th edition (DSM-IV). (American Psychiatric Association), 1994.

12. In a report entitled "Trends in the Prescribing of Psychotropic Medications to Preschoolers," *Journal of the American Medical Association* 283 (February 23, 2000): 1025-30, Zito, et al., confirm that "psychotropic medications prescribed for preschoolers increased dramatically between 1991 and 1995. The number of 2 to 4-year-olds on psychiatric drugs including Ritalin and antidepressants like Prozac soared 50 percent between 1991 and 1995. In an accompanying editorial Harvard's Dr. Joseph Coyle said "this study [Zito, et al.] reveals a troubling trend given that there is no empirical evidence to support psychotropic drug treatment in very young children and that there are valid concerns that such treatment could have deleterious effects on the developing brain. These disturbing prescription practices suggest a growing crisis in mental health services to children and demand more thorough investigation."

Chapter 4

1. Zito, et al., estimate that some 150,000-200,000 children between the ages of 2 and 4 in the United States are cur-

rently receiving prescriptions for methylphenidate—Ritalin See Huget, Jennifer. *Washington Post*, (January 2, 2001): T06. Steven E. Hyman, director of the National Institute of Mental Health (NIMH) asks: "How can we tolerate a situation in which drugs are prescribed to an increasing number of preschoolers without safety and efficacy data?" Moreover, and Hyman knows it, none of the preschoolers, toddlers and infants, thus-treated, in fact, no child of any age, given such psychiatric diagnoses, has any real disease. This should be the source of outrage, not that they have not undergone clinical trials of these drugs. Laurence Greenhill, of the New York State Psychiatric Institute, one of their own, answers, "We can't " [tolerate the lack of "safety and efficacy data."] . In turn, they organized a consortium of six academic departments of child-now-infant psychiatry to apply for a grant to study the effects of Ritalin on a group of children ranging in age from 3 to 6 years of age. The PATS research, they acknowledge, has raised ethical questions including whether children this young should be given Ritalin which clearly alters the way the brain works. But they said nothing about the most important objection of all: that the infants to be recruited as subjects are normal, that they have no identifiable disease, in fact that ADHD, regardless of the age, is not known to be a bona fide disease, one with a confirming, characteristic, objective abnormality. Their first and only abnormality will be the always brain-altering, brain-damaging Ritalin, Drs. Hyman and Greenhill and their collaborators intend to put them on.

2. Learning disabilities are claimed to be brain disorders/diseases to make normal children fodder for "special education" just as ADHD makes them fodder for drugging. Not even dyslexia has been validated as a disease. Seeking

246   THE ADHD FRAUD

to determine whether "discrepancy testing"—subtracting one's reading achievement score from one's IQ (aptitude)—reliably diagnoses "dyslexia." See Shaywitz, SE, et al. *New England Journal of Medicine* 326 (1992):145-150 who found that only 28% of the children identified as "dyslexic" in the first grade still had it in the third grade. They were forced to conclude: "This study allowed us to investigate the commonly held belief that dyslexia is a discrete diagnostic entity. Our data do not support this notion." [A roundabout way of saying it is not a disease.] Nor has an abnormality of the brain been found since. See Stanovich, KE in the *Journal of Child Psychology and Psychiatry* 35 (1994): 579-95, who observes: "The reading field seems unnaturally prone to popularizing terminology that carries with it unproven theory."

3. The June, 1, 1990 issue of *The Medical Letter on Drugs and Therapeutics* reported the sudden deaths of three children with "behavior disorders" taking the tricyclic antidepressant, desipramine. See "Sudden Death in children treated with a tricyclic antidepressant," p. 792-7. Next, came the 1993 report of a fourth sudden death with desipramine. See Riddle, MA, et al. "Another sudden death in a child treated with desipramine," *Journal of the American Academy of Child and Adolescent Psychiatry* 32 (1993): 792-7. Following the fourth death, the *Journal of the American Academy of Child and Adolescent Psychiatry* published a debate between child psychiatrists John Werry of the University of Auckland, New Zealand and Joseph Biederman of Harvard University and three of their colleagues who argue that desipramine "merely ameliorates," "does not cure" and "could never be described as life-saving." Werry argued that "pharmacologic and toxicological data, pragmatic and ethical considerations suggest that desipramine

should no longer be used clinically in children." What he neglected to say in portraying the risk/benefit ratio was that none of the behavioral disorders for which this drug is prescribed—ADHD, childhood depression, obsessive-compulsive and panic disorder, conduct and oppositional-defiant disorder are proven diseases, or anything whatsoever biologic or organic. Defending desipramine and urging its continued use, Beiderman dismisses as "anecdotal" the deaths of four children with no organic disease that occurred while those children were taking medication known to be heart-toxic. The only physical risk that these or any children similarly diagnosed are confronted with are those borne by the medications they are given. They had no "disease" to begin with, that is, at the time of diagnosis. See Werry, JS, Biederman, J, Thisted, R, Greenhill, L, and Ryan, N. "Resolved: cardiac arrhythmias make desipramine an unacceptable choice in children," *Journal of the American Academy of Child and Adolescent Psychiatry* 34 (1995):1239-45. As we know, desipramine remained available for use in child psychiatry and was the cause of death of 6 year old Shaina Dunkle in 2001.

4. What they don't tell you, most importantly, is that ADHD is not a disease, that no psychiatric disorder/illness/chemical imbalance/disease is an actual disease; that the first and only disease is the intoxication from the drug or drugs. The "disease" lie, in and of itself seduces parents into drugging/poisoning their own children while at the same time abrogating their right to informed consent. In the case of Shaina Dunkle, the disease lie led her parents, Vicki and Steve, to conclude that treatment was necessary and to go along with putting her on desipramine a drug whose contraindications precautions, adverse reactions, and signs of overdosage run 3 fine-print columns in

the PDR. She had no real disease to begin with, only the mounting risks of polypharmacy on the risk side of the risk vs. benefit equation.

5. See *Stedman's Medical Dictionary*, 25th edition (Williams and Wilkins, 1990).

6. Compare the real "chemical imbalances" described herein to the fraudulent, non-existent "chemical imbalances" of psychiatry—all of them bought, paid for, and legitimized by Congress and the White House. See "Inconsistencies in Screening Mean Rare Diseases Go Undetected and Untreated," *The Wall Street Journal* (June 17, 2004). Zachary Wyvill was born with a very rare enzyme deficiency that has left him unable to eat, walk or crawl. A month later, another child named Zachary was born with the same genetic disorder in a hospital 60 miles to the east. But today, this boy, Zachary Black is a healthy 1 year old. His disease is kept in check with a special diet and vitamins. His condition was diagnosed during a special newborn-screening project carried out in many, but not all, California hospitals. Zachary Wyville's condition wasn't detected because his blood wasn't screened. "By some government and medical estimates, the lack of standardized newborn screening is responsible for the illness and death of several thousand children every year. The cost of treating and caring for children who suffer from these rare diseases can range from $500,000 to $1 million according to the US Centers for Disease Control and Prevention (CDC). "No child in America with one of these diseases should ever go undetected at birth" says Harry Hannon, director of newborn-screening services at the CDC. Compare this to the monstrous, growing expenditures in the fraudulent marketplace of psychiatric diseases/chemical imbalances—none of them real. This fraudulent, absolutely unnec-

essary, spending is clearly a factor in rendering 45 million Americans unable to afford health care insurance.

7. See Bellanti, JA, et al. "Ataxia-telangiectasia: immunologic and virologic studies of serum and respiratory secretions," *Pediatrics* 37 (1966): 924.

8. Baughman, FA, Jr.: "CHANDS: The Curly Hair-Ankyloble-pharon-Nail Dysplasia Syndrome" in *The Clinical Delineation of Birth Defects*, v.12 (1972).

9. Toriello, HV, Lindstrom, JA., Waterman, DF., and Baughman, FA, Jr. "Re-Evaluation of CHANDS," *Journal of Medical Genetics* 16 (1979): 316.

10. Neurology deals with real diseases, psychiatry with emotions and behaviors. See *The American Academy of Neurology: The First 50 Years*, 1948-1998 (American Academy of Neurology): 1-8.

11. There is no such thing as a psychiatric disease. See Congressional Office of Technology Assessment. *The Biology of Mental Disorders* (US Government Printing Office, 1992): 13-14, 46-47.

Chapter 5

1. See *Diagnostic and Statistical Manual of Mental Disorders, 4th edition* (American Psychiatric Association, 1994)

2. "Attention-deficit/hyperactivity disorder is the most common neurobehavioral disorder of childhood." See Committee on Quality Improvement, Subcommittee on Attention-Deficit/Hyperactivity Disorder Guidelines of the American Academy of Pediatrics, "Clinical Practice Guideline: Diagnosis and Evaluation of the Child with Attention-Deficit/Hyperactiviity Disorder," *Pediatrics* 105 (2000):1158.

To which Baughman responded: "Neurobehavioral," implies an abnormality of the brain; a disease. And yet, no confirmatory, diagnostic, abnormality has been found. With six million children said to have it, most of them on addictive, dangerous, stimulants, ambiguity as to the scientific status of ADHD is not acceptable." "It is apparent that virtually all professionals of the extended ADHD 'industry' convey to parents, and to the public-at-large, that ADHD is a 'disease' and that children said to have it are 'diseased'-'abnormal.' This is a perversion of the scientific record and a violation of the informed consent rights of all patients and of the public-at-large. The wording of the AAP Guideline should be changed, forthwith, to reflect the scientific and medical facts of the matter" See Baughman, FA, Jr. "Diagnosis and Evaluation of the Child With Attention-Deficit/Hyperactivity Disorder," (letter) *Pediatrics* 107 (2001): 1239.

3. See Wasserman, RC, et al. "Identification of Attentional and Hyperactivity Problems in Primary Care: A report from Pediatric Research in Office Settings and the Ambulatory Sentinel Practice Network," *Pediatrics* 103 (March, 1999): e38.

4. See Granger, Lori and Bill. *The Magic Feather: the truth about special education.* (Dell, 1986).

5. The Council on Scientific Affairs of the American Medical Association concluded: "...there is little evidence of widespread over-diagnosis or misdiagnosis of ADHD or of widespread over-prescription of methylphenidate." See Goldman, LS et al. "Council on Scientific Affairs, American Medical Association. Treatment of Attention-Deficit/Hyperactivity Disorder," *JAMA* 279 (1998): 1100-07. Baughman responded: "Once children are labeled with ADHD, they are no longer treated as normal. Once

methylphenidate hydrochloride (Ritalin) or any psychotropic drug courses through their brain and body, they
are, for the first time, physically, neurologically and biologically abnormal." See Baughman, FA, Jr. *JAMA* 281
(1999):1490-91.

6. Kirk, S.A., and Kutchins, H. (1992). *The Selling of DSM:
The Rhetoric of Science in Psychiatry.* Hawthorne, New
York: Aldine de Gruyter.

7. "One in 14 men suffers from depression..." "Men need to
know depression is not a weakness but a treatable disease." "More than 6 million men in the US—one in every
14—suffer from this insidious disorder..." "Depression,
like heart disease, looks different in men than in women"
says Dr. Thomas Insel, director of the National Institute
of Mental Health. "If untreated, depression takes a toll
on the body as well as the brain... If you have depression,
it appears to increase your risk of getting heart disease,"
says Dr. Dennis Charney, head of the NIMH's research
program for depression and anxiety. "Depression is not a
weakness but a highly treatable medical disease," says Dr.
Richard Carmona, the US Surgeon General. See Hales,
Dianne and Robert. *Parade Magazine* (June 20, 2004).
Here we have depression, a ubiquitous, normal emotion—
regardless of severity—called a disease, and the current
Surgeon General, the leading government physician, a
party to the lie that holds that all things psychiatric are
diseases, when none are.

8. "Bipolar disorder is a chemical imbalance in the brain that
causes alternating episodes of mania and depression..."
See Papolos, Demitri. The Bipolar Child (Broadway
Books), quoted in the *San Diego Union-Tribune*, June 17,
2000: E-1. "Daniel's mother and tens of thousands of others across the country are latching on to a new diagnosis

...bipolar disorder or manic-depressive illness, a condition once thought to be as rare in childhood as Halley's Comet. Driving this new diagnostic frenzy is the desire to find a label for unmanageable children whose angry moods and erratic behavior go beyond the attention problems and excessive energy of a child with ADHD. The diagnostic shift from ADHD to 'bipolar' has been intensified by a book that came out earlier this year, *The Bipolar Child*. A heated debate in child psychiatry has emerged in the past few years over the bipolar label, and it's not just an argument over semantics. Harvard's Joseph Biederman, a leading proponent of the bipolar diagnosis, said, 'my academic colleagues say they have never seen a case of bipolar illness in childhood. We need scientific evidence to know what to call it and when to call it,' said Dr. Peter Jensen, chairman of child and adolescent psychiatry at Columbia University College of Physicians and Surgeons. See Talan, Jamie. "The Bipolar Shift: psychiatric diagnosis for adults is becoming a new way to explain kids' emotional and behavioral disorders" *San Diego Union-Tribune* (October 13, 2000): E1. The schism between Biederman and Jensen seems remarkable. How, if both were referring to the same scientific literature, the same body of research, could they harbor such disparate views? The answer is simple, there are no objective abnormalities, no bona fide diseases. Psychiatry is not science at all, everything is subjective. Kids Doctors should be careful in prescribing stimulants and antidepressants to hyperactive children, according to Catrien G. Reichart, MD, of the Academisch Ziekenhuis in Rotterdam, Netherlands. "The prevalence of bipolar disorder in adolescents is much greater for American children (39 percent) than for Dutch children (4 percent)." Dr. Reichart and colleagues studied children in the United States and the Netherlands who had a parent with bipolar disorder. Their results show that the prevalence of bipolar disorder in these at-risk adolescents is much greater for American children (39 percent) than for Dutch children (4 percent). In the Netherlands there were very few cases of bipolar disorder found in children younger than 20, while in the US, children younger than 12 had been diagnosed—a US phenomena. The difference, according to Dr. Reichart, may be due to the use of stimulants and antidepressants to treat American children with hyperactivity, while doctors in The Netherlands rely more on psychosocial approaches. What they are saying is that the drugs US kids are being put on—stimulants and antidepressants—are causing symptoms of bipolar disorder. See University of Pittsburgh Medical School, "US kids 10 times more likely to suffer bipolar; ADHD drugs blamed (June 14, 2001).

9. "Paxil, the most prescribed medication of its kind for generalized anxiety, works to correct the chemical imbalance believed to cause the disorder." See Special Advertising Feature, *Family Circle Magazine* (November 20, 2001).

Chapter 6

1. See Silver, Larry. *ADHD and Learning Disabilities: Booklet for the Classroom Teacher* (Learning Disabilities Association of America), 16 pp (two dollars).

2. Here we have an example of "government" in the big pharma-psychiatry-government, drugging triumvirate. Others abound, such as President Bush's New Freedom Commission on Mental Health, which seeks to implement mental health screening throughout the public schools of the nation. See *Attention Deficit Disorder: Beyond the Myths* (U.S. Department of Education, 1994).

3. Pittsburgh Modified Conners Teacher Rating Scale. See Conners, CK, et al. "The Revised Conners' Parent Rating Scale CPRS-R: factor structure, reliability, and criterion validity," *Journal of Abnormal Child Psychology* 26 (1998): 257-68.

4. See Attention-Deficit/Hyperactivity Disorder Test (AD-HDT) for the evaluation of attention-deficit disorders in persons 3-23(PRO-ED, 8700 Shoal Creek Blvd., Austin, TX, 78757-6897).

5. See Hallowell Index: 50 Tips on the Management of Attention Deficit Disorder in Adults (Adapted from *Driven to Distraction* by Hallowell and Ratey, 1994)

6. See Hallowell, EM and Ratey, JJ. *Driven To Distraction: Recognizing and Coping with Attention Deficit Disorder from Childhood through Adulthood* (Simon and Schuster, 1994).

7. See Anxiety Clinic of Temple University Adult Anxiety Checklist (Philadelphia, 2000-2001).

Chapter 7

1. See Wagner, KD, et al. "Efficacy of sertraline in the treatment of children and adolescents with major depressive disorder: two randomized controlled trials," *JAMA* 290 (August 27, 2003): 1033-41.

2. See Healy, David. *Let Them Eat Prozac* (New York University Press, 2004).

3. See Healy, David. *The Creation of Psychopharmacology.* (Harvard University Press, 2002).

4. "As more children pop pills for attention deficit and other behavior disorders, new figures show spending on those drugs has for the first time edged out the cost of antibiotics and asthma medications for kids. A 49 percent rise in the use of attention deficit/hyperactivity disorder drugs by children under 5 in the past three years contributed to a 23 percent increase in usage for all children, according to an analysis of drug trends by Medco Health Solutions Inc." See Johnson, Linda A. "Behavior drugs top kids' prescriptions. More spent than on antibiotics, asthma therapy," Trenton, NJ, *Associated Press*, (May 17, 2004). With 43 million US citizens without health care insurance —82 million without coverage for at least one month of the year—we have ADHD—an invented, contrived, fraudulent disease/epidemic having become one of the big-ticket items on the US health care budget.

5. Editor, Marcia Angell, MD, of the *New England Journal of Medicine* was surprised to learn that authors of an editorial favorable to obesity drug, Redux that appeared in the *Journal* (August 28, 1996) were paid consultants to firms making and marketing the drug. The editorial accompanied an article linking appetite suppressants, such as Redux, to a fatal lung disorder: pulmonary hypertension. The editorial argued that such drugs (Redux) could save 280 lives (lost due to obesity) for every 14 who die from the rare lung disorder (pulmonary hypertension). The lead author of the editorial, Harvard Associate Professor, JoAnn E. Manson, MD was a paid consultant for Interneuron in 1995, during the FDA review of the drug. Gerald A. Faich, MD, adjunct professor at the University of Pennsylvania testified before the FDA in 1995 as a paid consultant for Serview, the French company marketing the drug abroad. Faich, like most in medical academia caught with their

hand in the pot, rebutted: "My views are mine, they are independent; they are not biased by the source of funding." As word of the editorial leaked, Aug 27, Interneuron's stock rose 13% on Nasdaq. See Manson, J and Faich, G. "Pharmacotherapy for Obesity-Do the Benefits Outweigh the Risks?," *New England Journal of Medicine* 335 (August 29, 1996): 659-60 quoted in the *American Medical News* (October 7, 1996).

6. See Whittington, CJ, et al. "Selective serotonin reuptake inhibitors in childhood depression: systematic review of published versus unpublished data," *Lancet* 363 (9418) April 24, 2004:1341-45.

7. "Depressing Research" (editorial). *Lancet* 363 (9418) April 24, 2004: 1335.

8. See Baumeister, AA and Hawkins, MF. "Incoherence of neuroimaging studies of attention deficit/hyperactivity disorder," *Clinical Neuropharmacology* 24 (2001): 2-10.

9. See Zametkin, AJ, et al. "Cerebral Glucose Metabolism in Adults with Hyperactivity of Childhood Onset (a positron emission tomography-PET scan study)," *New England. Journal of Medicine* 323 (1990): 1361-66.

10. Functional MRI (fMRI) scans show which areas of the normal brains are functioning during certain activities—speech, moving a thumb, leg, arm; which parts of the brain "light up" in certain moods, postures, etc. Psychiatry claims that the functional-MRI correlates of various moods, such as depression, anxiety, panic, define a disease, when it does not and cannot. Structural, also known as anatomic MRI (sMRI) scans are in routine use in neurology to diagnose real diseases such as tumors, strokes, multiple sclerosis, traumatic brain injuries and brain atrophy, such

as that caused by Ritalin/amphetamine treatment, visible by CT or MRI scan, to the naked eye.

11. See Nasrallah, HA, et al. "Cortical atrophy in young adults with a history of hyperactivity in childhood," *Psychiatric Research* 17 (1986): 241-46.

12. See Swanson, J. and Castellanos, FX. *NIH Consensus Development Conference on ADHD: Biological Bases of Attention Deficit Hyperactivity Disorder* (NIH, November 16-18, 1998): 37-42.

13. See Hynd, GW, et al. "Brain morphology in developmental dyslexia and attention deficit disorder/hyperactivity," *Archives of Neurology* 47 (1990): 919-26.

14. See Hynd, GW, et al. "Corpus callosum morphology in attention-deficit hyperactivity disorder: morphometric analysis of MRI," *Journal of Learning Disabilities* 24 (1991): 141-46.

15. See Hynd, GW, et al. "Attention deficit hyperactivity disorder and asymmetry of the caudate nucleus," *Journal of Child Neurology* 8 (1993):339-47.

16. See Giedd, JN, et al. "Quantitative morphology of the corpus callosum in attention deficit hyperactivity disorder," *American Journal of Psychiatry* 151 (1994): 665-69.

17. Castellanos, FX, et al. "Quantitative morphology of the caudate nucleus in attention deficit hyperactivity disorder," *American Journal of Psychiatry* 151 (1994): 1791-96.

18. See Semrud-Clikeman, M, et al. "Attention-deficit hyperactivity disorder: magnetic resonance imaging morphometric analysis of the corpus callosum," *Journal of the American Academy of Child and Adolescent Psychiatry* 33 (1994): 875-81.

19. See Baumgardner, TL, et al. "Corpus callosum morphology in children with Tourette syndrome and attention deficit hyperactivity disorder," *Neurology* 47 (1996): 477-82.

20. See Aylward, EH, et al. "Basal ganglia volumes in children with attention-deficit hyperactivity disorder," *Journal of Child Neurology* 11 (1996): 112-15.

21. See Castellanos, FX, et al. "Quantitative brain magnetic resonance imaging in attention-deficit/hyperactivity disorder," *Archives of General Psychiatry* 53 (1996): 607-16.

22. See Filipek, PA, et al. "Volumetric MRI analysis comparing attention-deficit hyperactivity disorder and normal controls," *Neurology* 48 (1997): 589-601.

23. See Casey, BJ, et al. "Implication of right frontostriatal circuitry in response inhibition and attention-deficit/hyperactivity disorder," *Journal of the American Academy of Child and Adolescent Psychiatry* 36 (1997): 374-83.

24. See Mataro, M, et al. "Magnetic resonance imaging measurement of the caudate nucleus in adolescents with attention-deficit hyperactivity disorder and its relationship with neuropsychological and behavioral measures," *Archives of Neurology* 54 (1997): 963-68.

25. See Berquin, PC, et al. "The cerebellum in attention-deficit/hyperactivity disorder: a morphometric study," *Neurology* 50 (1998): 1087-93.

26. See Mostofsky, SH, et al. "Evaluation of cerebellar size in attention-deficit hyperactivity disorder," *Journal of Child Neurology* 13 (1998): 434-39.

27. Two of these studies did not report whether the ADHD subjects were medicated or not and one did not report clearly. Leo and Cohen estimate that 247 of the 259 to-

tal ADHD subjects in these studies —95%—had been medicated (ADHD-medicated). See Leo, JL and Cohen, DA. "Broken brains or flawed studies? A critical review of ADHD neuroimaging studies," *The Journal of Mind and Behavior* 24 (2003): 29-56.

28. This wording appeared in the version of the final statement of the CC Panel distributed at the press conference, the final session of the CC, November, 18, 1998. An indeterminate few months later, it was removed from the NIH website and replaced with wording claiming 'validity' for ADHD.

29. A January, 2000, *Reader's Digest* article reported: "Castellanos and his group found three areas of the brain to be significantly smaller in ADHD kids than in normal children...Some critics claim that such brain differences in ADHD children might actually be caused by Ritalin...To address this, Castellanos has now embarked on another study, imaging the brains of ADHD youngsters who have not been treated with drugs." See Pekkanen, J. "Making Sense of Ritalin (interview of F.X. Castellanos)," *Readers Digest* (January, 2000):159-68

30. See Castellanos, FX, et al. "Developmental Trajectories of Brain Volume Abnormalities in Children and Adolescents With Attention–Deficit/Hyperactivity Disorder," *JAMA* 288 (2002): 1740-48.

31. Bartzokis G, et al. "Brain maturation may be arrested in chronic cocaine addicts." *Biological Psychiatry* 15 (2002): 605-611.

32. See Sowell, et al. "Cortical abnormalities in children and adolescents with attention-deficit hyperactivity disorder," *The Lancet* 363 (2003):1699-1707.

33. See Leo, JL and Cohen, DA. "Broken brains or flawed studies? A critical review of ADHD neuroimaging studies," *The Journal of Mind and Behavior* 24 (2003): 29-56.

Chapter 8

1. Rezulin, a diabetes drug, caused 61 deaths before it was taken off of the market. It took a FDA physician going directly to members of Congress to get the FDA to act. The British government took it off the market a long time ago. See Manning, Anita. *USA Today* (March 23, 2000).

2. See Kuttner, Robert *The San Diego Union–Tribune* (June 29, 1998).

3. Unlike Britain's Medicines and Healthcare Products Regulatory Agency which recently warned doctors against prescribing any SSRI antidepressant except Prozac for youths, a group called the American College of Neuropsychopharmacology has come to the conclusion that Prozac and all of its SSRI relatives, Paxil, Zoloft, Luvox, Celexa, etc., should remain in use to treat "clinically" depressed youngsters, calling evidence linking the drugs to suicidal behavior weak. See Patterson, Karen. "Group endorses use of anti-depressants in teens," *The Dallas Morning News* (January 21, 2004).

4. Stubbe DE, Thomas WJ. "A Survey of Early-career Child and Adolescent Psychiatrists: Professional Activities and Perceptions", *Journal of the American Academy of Child and Adolescent Psychiatry* 2002 Feb; 41(2):123-30.

5. See DEA Drug Enforcement Administration of the US Department of Justice, Drug and Chemical Evaluation Section, Office of Diversion Control. *Methylphenidate : a background paper* (October, 1995).

6. Lambert, N and Hartsough, CS. "Prospective study of tobacco smoking and substance dependence among samples of ADHD and non-ADHD subjects," *Journal of Learning Disabilities* 31 (1998): 533-44.

Chapter 9

1. See Jensen, Peter. "Opposing View," *USA Today* (August 15, 2000): 16A.

2. See Carey, William, MD and McDevitt, Sean, PhD. *Coping with Children's Temperament* (Basic Books, 1995).

Chapter 10

1. Daniel R Weinberger, MD, Chief of the Clinical Brain Disorders Branch of the National Institute of Mental Health, explained that neuroimaging in the form of MRI (magnetic resonance imaging), fMRI (functional- magnetic resonance imaging), and PET (positron emission tomography) has demonstrated that most major psychiatric disease—depressive disorders and schizophrenia, for example—are associated with "subtle but objectively characterizable changes" in brain structure and function. "These changes do not establish the diagnosis but do demonstrate the involvement of the brain in these disorders" See McBride, G. "Neuroimaging Advances Offer New Data on Stroke Detection and the Genetics of Mental Illness," *Neurology Today* (June, 2002): 26-8. Subsequently, I wrote the editor of *Neurology Today* stating: "Dr. Weinberger must submit for publication in *Neurology Today*, references for the claim that "neuroimaging in the form of MRI, fMRI, and PET has demonstrated that most major psychiatric disease—depressive disorders and schizophrenia, for example—are associated with "subtle but objectively char-

acterizable changes" in brain structure and function." If he is unable to present proof of the "subtle but objectively characterizable changes" in these psychiatric conditions, the editors of should say so and print a retraction." Here, Dr. Weinberger, speaking for all of US psychiatry claimed there were "subtle but objectively characterizable changes" without giving references to any such proofs in the scientific literature. Nor has *Neurology Today*, its editor, or the American Academy of Neurology (AAN) retracted these statements.

2. In August, 2003, hunger strikers from Mindfreedom-Support Coalition International (of which I am a member and scientific advisor) wrote to the American Psychiatric Association (APA) asking for proof that psychiatric "diseases" are actual abnormalities/diseases. On Friday, September 26, 2003, the APA released its Statement on Diagnosis and Treatment of Mental Disorders, which stated: "Over the past five years, the nation has more than doubled its investment in the study of the human brain and behavior leading to a vastly expanded understanding of disorders that afflict and are mediated by the brain." Here, they failed, once more, to define what they mean by "disorders" and anticipate we could never imagine that they would spend so much money on research on things never proved to actual diseases. In fact, the "research" which we fund (through taxes), and they perform, creates illusions of diseases—which psychiatry, then, diagnoses and treats. The APA: " It is unfortunate that in the face of this remarkable scientific and clinical progress, a small number of individuals and groups persist in questioning the reality and clinical legitimacy of disorders that affect the mind, brain, and behavior. One recent challenge contended that the lack of a diagnostic

laboratory test capable of confirming the presence of a
mental disorder constituted evidence that these disorders
are not medically valid conditions." By "disorder" psychiatry means disease (disease = abnormality). This is
what all physicians who practice "biological" psychiatry
and "biological" mental health tell their patients and the
public. This is the "big lie!"   Nowhere in their Statement
on Diagnosis and Treatment of Mental Disorders, did
the APA cite a proof that ADHD or any single, psychiatric condition/disorder/chemical imbalance is an actual
disease. In responding to Support Coalition, the APA
referred them to a short list of psychiatric textbooks, just
as Dr. Weinberger had done in writing to me—confes-
sions that there are no articles in the scientific literature,
proving that any such thing as a psychiatric abnormal-
ity/disease/disorder/chemical imbalance, really exists.

3. See Werner, Erica. "Mentally Ill Youths 'Warehoused'," *Associated Press*, Washington, D.C., (July 8, 2004).

4. See Lenzer, Jeanne. "Bush plans to screen whole US population for mental illness," *BMJ* 328 (2004): 1458.

Index

Acupuncture, 213

Adderall, 5, 31, 42, 76, 142–43, 168, 169, 177, 196, 197, 198, 231

  Withdrawal of, 227

Alpert, Bernard, 188

American Academy of Child and Adolescent Psychiatry, 6

American Psychiatric Association (APA), 6, 69, 116, 178

American Society of Adolescent Psychiatry, 26, 186

Amphetamines, 2, 52-54, 180, 234m

Anthony, Susan B., 63

Antidepressants. See SSRI

Attention deficit disorder (ADD), 9, 30, 31, 54, 55, 69-70, 92

Attention deficit hyperactivity disorder (ADHD)

  Common diagnostic practices, 4, 16, 20, 24, 27-28, 34-35, 58, 74, 116, 122, 158

  Complicity of schools in identifying, 13, 145, 178

Criteria for diagnosing, 104–06

Diagnosis of, 9, 16, 30, 31, 33–4, 122, 178

American Medical Association agreement with, 118–19

Evidence supporting diagnosis for, 180–83

Genetic etiology for, 179

Hyperactive child syndrome, precursor to, 29

Lack of medical evidence for, 6, 92–3, 158

Labeling of child for, 3, 4, 58, 220, 224

Lifetime affliction, 159–64

MRI (Magnetic Resonance Imaging) and, 180, 184–86, 257m

  Noncompliance of children as reason for, 24, 34, 191

  Non-disease status of, 8–9, 13, 17, 74, 92–4, 120–21, 142–43, 159, 179, 206–07, 210–11, 225, 237n, 248n, 249n, 263n

  Non-prescribed use of, 240m

Prescribed drugs for, 5, 14–5, 42, 45, 54, 169–70, 213, 220

Personal accounts

Adam, 14–16

Cameron, 43–44, 200

Chris, 18–20

Daniel, 196–98

Duane, 29–30

Kara, 193

Kyle, 25–27

Matthew, 1–9

Max, 35–39

Michael, 48–50

Paul, 40–43

Rod, 239m

Ryan, 240m

Shaina, 44, 78–85, 200

Stephanie, 9–13

Youngs, 67–69

Research for, 178–86

Subtests for, 153–60

Subtypes of, 114–16

Attention Deficit Hyperactivity Disorder, Combined Type

Attention Deficit Hyperactivity Disorder, Predominately Inattentive Type

Attention Deficit Hyperactivity Disorder, Predominately Hyperactive-Impulsive Type

Attention Deficit Hyperactivity Disorder Not Otherwise Specified

Symptoms of, 71, 122

Test for, 153–55

Barkley, Russell, 33

Behavior modifying drugs, 47

Beneficiaries of prescribing, 45–46, 56, 61–62, 64, 65, 76, 161

Benzedrine, 53–54

Biofeedback, 213

Bipolar disorder, 20, 130–36, 197, 251–53n

Bradley, Charles, 52–54

Brain atrophy, 180, 182–85, 208, 229

Breggin, Peter, 7

Burke, James Lee, 44

Caplan, Arthur, 194

Carey, William, 39, 45–46, 58, 59, 121, 215, 219

Castellanos, F. Xavier, 180, 181, 183, 184, 185, 186, 208

Cartwright, Samuel and 19th century diagnosing, 176–77

CHADD (Children and Adults with Attention Deficit Disorders), 140, 142

Chiropractic, 213

Clarke, Arthur C., 126

Clonidine, 14

Cocaine, 2, 76, 119, 195

Collins, Susan, 220

Concerta, 15, 144, 227

Conduct Disorder, 122–25

Coyle, Joseph, 72, 244m

Cylert, 42, 233

DARE (Drug Abuse Resistance Education) program, 64, 75–76

Degrandpre, Richard, 75

Depakote, 42, 177

Depression, 20, 127, 163–64, 251m

Desipramine (antidepressant), 43, 44, 78, 81–84, 200

Dexedrine, 5, 14, 41, 54, 168

Diagnostic and Statistical Manual of Mental Disorders (DSM), 45, 69–73, 102–03, 156, 242–44m

Diller, Lawrence, 39, 44, 192

Diminishment of child, 114

Disease, definition of, 58–59, 86–95, 243–46m

Disruptive Behavior Disorder Not Otherwise Specified, 123

Drug Enforcement Administration (DEA), 2, 31, 39

Dyslexia, 245–246m

Dysthymic disorder, 129–30

Elliot, Carl, 165

Food and Drug Administration (FDA), 8, 55, 57, 174, 192, 195, 227, 229, 230

Fukuyama, Francis, 16, 17

Gallagher, Cornelius (Gallagher Report), 52, 60, 61–64, 66–67, 74

Garland, Jane, 172

Generalized Anxiety Disorder, 136–37

Glenmullen, Joseph, 175

Granger, Lori and Bill, 117–18

Griffith, John, 52, 221–222

Haldol, 179

Hallowell, Edward, 159, 178

Hallowell Index, 159

Haslip, Gene, 32, 33

Healy, David, 42, 54, 57, 60, 140, 166, 196

Health Canada, 226

Holt, John, 64–66

House Education Committee, 4

Huxley, Aldous, 204

Hyperactivity, 110

Hyperkinetic reaction (early diagnostic term for ADHD), 55

Informed consent, 94, 200–02, 211–13, 222, 229–31, 235m

Jensen, Peter, 32, 203

Jung, Carl, 118

Keller, Martin, 166

Kendall, Tim, 172, 173

Kessler, David, 195

Kirk, Stuart, 121

Koplewicz, Harold, 73, 208

Kutchins, Herb, 121

Leber, Paul, 229

Lewis, C.S., 21

Major Depressive Disorder, Single Episode, 127–29

McDevitt, Sean, 58, 59

McGuinness, Diane, 27

Medicalizing of human life, 57, 99, 177–78, 207

Merton, Thomas, 46

Minimal brain dysfunction (precursor to ADD), 55–56, 62, 64, 68, 69

Mosher, Loren, 75

Mosholder, Andrew, 174

National Commission on Excellence in Education, 118

National Institutes of Health, 17, 121

National Institute of Mental Health, 60, 178, 185

Neurontin, 169, 177

New Freedom Commission on Mental Health, 221, 253m

Newman, Nathan, 165

NIH Consensus Conference on ADHD, 45–46, 121

Obetrol (prior trade name of Ritalin), 31–32

Obsessive Compulsive Disorder, 137–39

Oppositional Defiant Disorder. See Conduct Disorder

Pelham, William, 227

Peters, John, 62

Pharmaceutical industry

Direct-to-consumer advertising, 170

Drug trials, 190–94

Influence of, 140, 173–74

Marketing by, 165–72, 174

Sales of ADHD drugs, 168, 169–71, 255

Pittsburgh Modified Conners Teacher Rating Scale, 146–52

Polypharmacy, 197–98, 212

Prescribing, off-label, 74

Prescription drugs for ADHD (psychiatric drugs), list of, 199–201

Toxicity of, 143, 200–201, 222–25

Prozac, 166–67, 176, 192, 195–96, 244

Psychiatry, role of, 98, 194

Risperdal, 42, 43, 178

Ritalin (methylphenidate), 1–2, 6-7, 10, 32, 62, 168, 182–83

Adverse effects of, 8, 10–11, 13, 18–19, 41, 185, 186, 194–95, 230

Approval by FDA, 57

Encephalopathy and, 212

Heart damage from, 1–2, 12, 230–31, 234–35

Prescription increase for, 32 33, 57, 65, 72, 121, 245n, 245–46n

Reports of death from, 228

Rosemond, John, 6

Seroquel, 42, 43

Silber, John, 120

Silver, Larry, 141

Social Anxiety Disorder, 161–64

SSRI (Selective Serotonin Reuptake Inhibitor), 171–76, 193, 200, 233

Celexa, 171, 192

Effexor, 171, 193

Paxil, 161, 162, 171, 192, 193,

Zoloft, 171, 192, 194–95

Still, George, 55

Stimulants, 2, 6, 76

Prescriptions for ADHD, 30–31

Strattera, 145, 170, 228

Swanson, James, 26, 181, 182, 186

Swift, Jonathan, 102

Szasz, Thomas, 100

Teacher Deficit Disorder (TDD), 59

Temperament (personality), 215–17

Thalidomide, 232

Thorazine, 178

Tofranil (antidepressant), 42

Tolstoy, Leo, 188

Wagner, Karen Dineen, 165–66

Waxman, Henry, 220

Wellbutrin, 42, 80, 197

Werry, John, 200

World Health Organization, 196

Yale University study, 20

Zeidner, Daniel, 59

Zyprexa, 197